Penguin Books
Dance Now

Jan Murray was born in Nova Scotia, Canada, and now
lives in London, though she travels throughout the world to
watch and report on dance. Two recent assignments have
taken her to Greece and India. After university in first
Canada and then the United States, she attended the Royal
Academy of Dramatic Art in London. She now works as
dance editor of London's *Time Out* magazine and dance
critic of the *Spectator*, and is a member of both the Dance
Committee of the Arts Council of Great Britain and the
Dance Panel of the Greater London Arts Association. *Dance
Now* is her first book.

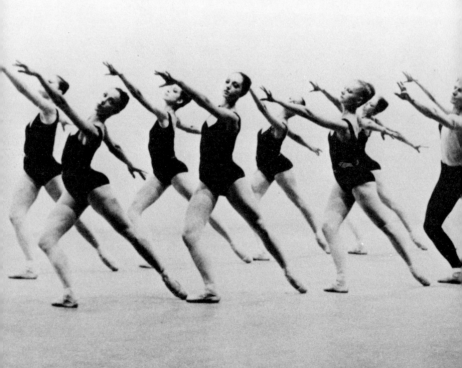

JAN MURRAY

Dance Now

PENGUIN BOOKS

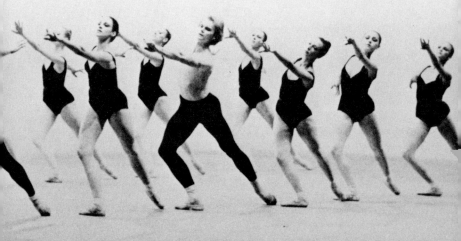

Penguin Books Ltd, Harmondsworth,
Middlesex, England
Penguin Books, 625 Madison Avenue,
New York, New York 10022, U.S.A.
Penguin Books Australia Ltd, Ringwood,
Victoria, Australia
Penguin Books Canada Ltd, 2801 John Street,
Markham, Ontario, Canada L3R 1B4
Penguin Books (N.Z.) Ltd, 182–190 Wairau Road,
Auckland 10, New Zealand

Published in Penguin Books 1979
Published simultaneously by Kestrel Books

Made and printed in Great Britain by
Richard Clay (The Chaucer Press) Ltd, Bungay, Suffolk
Set in 'Monophoto' Ehrhardt

Contents

Introduction

When I feel particularly gloomy or cheerful, or am afflicted by writer's block, I dance: all by myself, if necessary. It provides an amazing release, even though a detached observer might be somewhat jolted by the mixture of ballet, modern, tap and disco steps that emerges. The mixture stems from my own dance background; the impulse to move at such times is inherent in everyone.

Which is one reason I wrote this book. Dance, dancers and dancing have given me so much stimulation, challenge and joy that I have become a propagandist for the art – and the practice. Even today, when professional dance commands what is referred to as a 'mass audience', estimated in the USA alone at fifteen million, too many young people still associate professional dance with élitist culture or, more simply, think it has no relevance to their lives.

It does, if only because to live is to move, and the more freedom we have in movement, the more enjoyment we derive from watching highly trained bodies, the richer our existence becomes. To give a very personal example: when I was thirteen I had reached something close to my adult height of 5 ft 10 in. (1·75 m). The few girlfriends who suffered from a similar affliction tended to stoop, to back into corners at socials, to shy away from any activity that involved contact with boys (who were generally shorter, at that age) or public exposure. I had been studying ballet for five years by then, and however much I wanted to cower, I couldn't. Ballet is based on vertical line, on

7

elegance, on studied grace. I was unable to ignore all those sessions of concentrated training, even if I felt like cutting off my legs at the knee on occasion.

So I played basketball, I cheer-led (North American athletes could barely get through a game without the support of enthusiastic gymnasts on the sidelines), swam in competitions, indulged in figure-skating and horseback riding, until I was warned that those latter activities would develop the 'wrong' muscles for ballet. And I went to high school 'hops' and swooned over Elvis Presley and practised all the new jive steps with my buddies, in preparation for the next party. A normal teenager, though rather wholesome by today's less inhibited standards.

But I was determined that, somehow, I would become a professional dancer. Visions of myself as Giselle fluttered through my head, while I kept on growing. And what ballet company anywhere could provide a partner for a woman who loomed at six feet plus in point shoes? I knew something about modern dance, through a couple of mediocre films, but also knew that it was impossible to study 'barefoot techniques' seriously outside major American cities like New York or Los Angeles. And I lived in Nova Scotia, Canada.

I mention all this, not because my life has been marred by failure to achieve a youthful ambition, but because I want readers to understand how many more opportunities now exist for watching, studying and performing dance. Every kind of dance. (My home town of Halifax, Nova Scotia, now boasts a professional modern dance company, a number of different dance schools and frequent visits from world-famous troupes – and Halifax is not a large or central place.)

Discos can be a great training ground. So, for that matter, can listening to Bach and tracing out the formal patterns of his music in movement. So too *t'ai chi*, with its deep control and stillness; or contact improvisation, in which you roll over your partner like a friendly puppy; or an Indian classical dance style that develops parts of your body you didn't know existed; or an informal folk dance where you jig and bounce and swing and have a happy, sociable time.

And why not? Dance is about movement and can be an art, but it's also about communication – with yourself, as much as with other people. Dance is not effete or silly or overly refined – not often, at least. It is basic and we all do it, though we may call it 'body-language'.

I've been dancing and watching dance for more than twenty years, now. I never cease to learn from both processes. The blistered toes of my ballet days and the aching stomach muscles of my contemporary dance days (later on, in New York and London) have left me with a recognition of just how marvellous it is to feel your own body and to use it consciously as an instrument of expression. Maybe you're trying to work out some problem you can't put into words, or looking at a dancer who suddenly makes a gesture that strikes home. You experience an empathy, an understanding, that can only come through movement.

In this book I've tried to encapsulate the varied ways of achieving such an experience. This is not an academic, detailed history: simply a survey of where dance is now, and key figures who helped to provide the current range of dance techniques and philosophies. I've also given guidelines to studying dance, whether for fun, or for a professional stage or teaching career. The reference section at the back lists sources of research for the reader who wants to know more about some particular aspect of the art, with the emphasis on paperback books.

I wanted, too, to convey appreciation of the marvellous multiplicity of dance: the sweaty immediacy of punk Pogo; the sumptuous formality of Kabuki; the gut-twitching truth of contemporary styles; the cool beauty of classical ballet; the new vistas being opened by the best of the experimentalists. Some or all of these approaches are available to everyone, if only secondhand on television or in the cinema.

I owe an enormous debt to choreographers, musicians, designers, critics and, above all, performers, who have helped to make dance an integral part of my life. And as we must all begin somewhere, I must also pay tribute to my first teacher, a wonderful Latvian ballerina named Irene Apinee, who instilled in me a love of the art which continued after I had given up any idea of performing.

1·Mass Movements

Ours is a body-conscious age. With the increasing awareness of the need for physical exercise, we are regularly urged to 'move it'. The emphasis is on participation, for health and for creativity, so the millions of spectators who passively watch sports or, more recently, theatrical dance, are being countered by millions struggling to keep fit and express themselves through some kind of coordinated movement.

Styles and techniques have become universal. Westerners study karate and yoga, orientals have developed a passion for table tennis and classical ballet, while young people everywhere bop and grind out a form of social dance which stems from African tribal culture – rock. Everywhere there is an increasing interest in the needs and pleasures of the body and its art form, the dance.

In the opening scenes of the 1956 film *Rock around the Clock* an agent looks around a near empty commercial ballroom and declares, 'People aren't dancing any more, they're just listening. Big band business is dead.' Having sorted that out, he wanders off to a country town and there discovers Bill Haley and the Comets, the music group that is to awaken first America, then the world, to the phenomenon called rock'n'roll.

This screenplay, however corny, adhered closely to the facts. Haley's sound, with its all-pervasive pounding beat, may have been a pallid imitation of American Negro blues. Certainly his star was eclipsed within months by the emergence of Elvis 'the Pelvis' Presley. Yet it was the hit record *Rock around the Clock*, of which some fifteen million copies were sold, that zapped

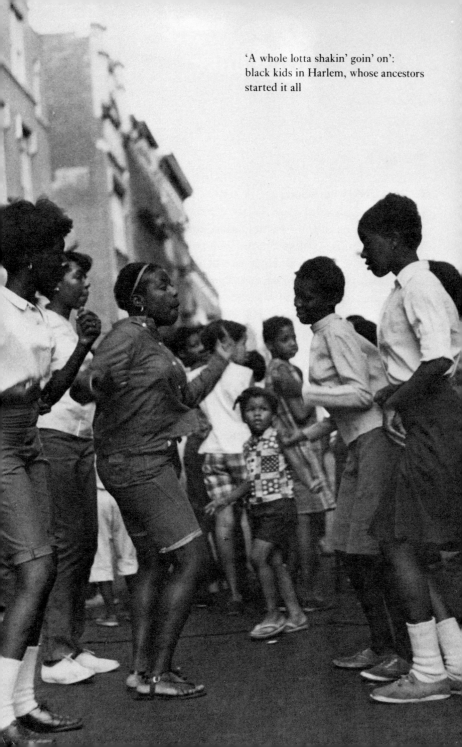

'A whole lotta shakin' goin' on':
black kids in Harlem, whose ancestors
started it all

teenagers back on to the dance floor. Suddenly, as a song of the fifties had it, there was 'a whole lotta shakin' goin' on'.

Rock'n'roll was only the latest, albeit the most popular, of recurring dance crazes which have swept across the west throughout modern history, beginning with the Waltz in 1814. An observer of that time noted, 'The people here [in Bavaria, Germany] are excessively fond of the pleasure of dancing; they need only hear the music of a waltz to begin to caper, no matter where they are ... Here we see artisans, merchants, councillors, barons, counts and excellencies dancing together with waitresses, women of the middle class, and ladies.' Ignoring traditional inhibitions, the hypnotic triple rhythm and the unusually intimate position of the couple, clasped in each other's arms, kept society whirling around for close to a century.

Then the influence of the 'New' World began to make itself felt – specifically, the black New World. A rhythmic complexity, freedom and sensuality were gradually injected into patterns of social dancing, and have remained to this day.

African slaves borrowed dance steps from their European masters, fused them with their own rich heritage, and evolved exciting new styles that were quickly taken up by whites. The first such creation was the Tango, and by the time Rudolph Valentino slunk elegantly through his own version in *The Four Horsemen of the Apocalypse* in 1921, Latin American dances were flooding the scene. Skill in interpreting the Rumba, the Samba, the Merenque or the Pasodoble became a guarantee of social acceptance. The famous exhibition dancers Vernon and Irene Castle demonstrated a more refined approach and, in their instruction manual, tried to turn the tide away from erotic movements, favouring politer forms like the Foxtrot. They warned: 'Do not wriggle the shoulders. Do not shake the hips. Do not twist the body. Drop the Turkey Trot, the Grizzly Bear, the Bunny Hug, etc. These dances are ugly, ungraceful and out of fashion.'

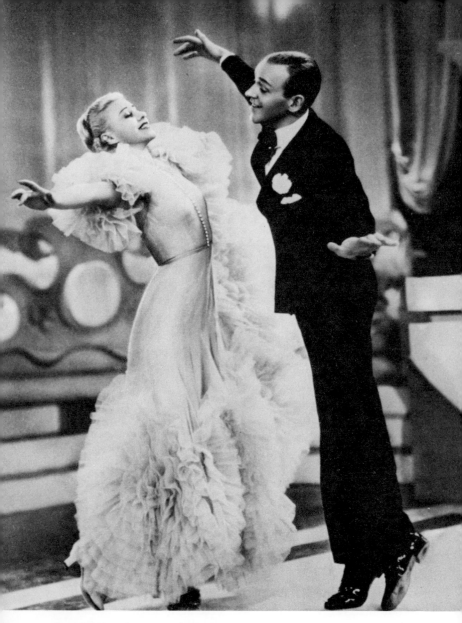

Fred Astaire, the master of effortless virtuosity in the ballroom and on the screen, with Ginger Rogers in the 1934 film, *Swing Time*

Too late. Already people were beginning to learn even more flamboyant styles of dancing, inspired by the indigenous black American music called jazz. Flappers of the twenties wriggled and bounced the Charleston, the Shimmy or the Black Bottom, and blithely ignored outraged accusations of vulgarity from the press. The dance marathons of the Depression, recorded in all their brutality by a recent film *They Shoot Horses, Don't They?*, set the seal on the dancing madness which galvanized the USA. It was at one such competition that George 'Shorty' Snowden contributed a major innovation to popular dance, the 'breakaway'.

This particular marathon went on for eighteen days, the contestants dancing around the clock (there was a fifteen-minute interval after each hour of dancing) until the New York Board of Health forcibly closed it down. On his way to winning a quarter of the $5,000 prize money, Snowden had tried to vary the monotony by breaking away from his partner and improvising his own solo steps. This seemingly minor variation, in what Snowden called the 'Lindy', led to a whole new approach to dancing. The writing was on the wall for the conventional couple arrangement; dancers began to do 'their own thing'.

The Lindy was the precursor of the modern styles that came to be collectively termed rock. It was sexy and smoothly violent, reflecting the tensions of that grim period. Young blacks like 'Shorty' Snowden burned up their nervous energy and frustrations by appearing almost every night in the famous Harlem dance halls. An unspoken rule among the regulars prevented people from copying anyone else's steps, so invention flourished. The big bands played fast, driving jazz and the dancers echoed the musical riffs and extemporizations with fresh, spontaneous movements. They danced on the floor and in the air, incorporated ju-jitsu and gymnastics, flung their partners around their hips or high over their heads, pulled them through their legs and bent them double.

By the time clarinettist Benny Goodman ushered in the

'swing era' of the thirties, the Lindy was known as the Jitterbug and had become established throughout America. The dancing uniform consisted of flat-heeled shoes, often saddle shoes, for both sexes, baggy trousers topped by long jackets for the men, full skirts that allowed the women to hurl themselves into athletic gyrations with complete abandon. Even these sloppy clothes could not conceal the vigorous movements of the hips and pelvis. Black sensuality had overwhelmed white repressions.

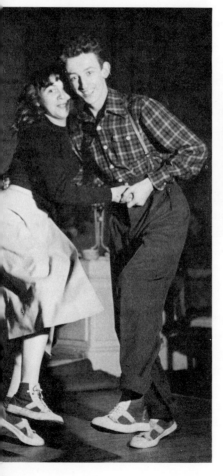

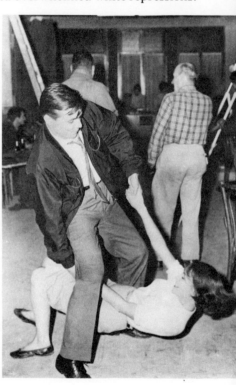

The Jitterbug, with participants sensibly dressed to allow maximum gyration

People still danced in couples, but they met and moved through different stages of rough contact, linking hands at arms' length. This, too, reflected the African influence, for in those Negro cultures where dance pervaded every area of life, body contact was avoided. Although Afro-Americans copied European footwork on occasion, they retained their traditional posture – a fluid spine and flexed knees, with the motion beginning in the centre of the body and rippling through to the head and limbs. Emerging in some dances were elements of mime and animal imitations, witness the modern Hitch Hike or the Chicken. Above all, the black dances were characterized by dominating, percussive rhythms. Originally these were played on drums, but when the volume of the beat became amplified by the new-fangled electric guitar, popular dancing lost the last traces of sedateness and conscious control.

But first the Jitterbug had to be exported across the Atlantic. American G Is serving in the Second World War took care of that, and the British, in particular, responded with alacrity to what they called Jiving. After the war this enthusiasm began to wane, however, as jazz musicians, led by experimentalists like Charlie 'Bird' Parker, turned to Bop, with its intricate, undanceable rhythms, and ballad singers like Frank Sinatra became all the rage.

In his book *Awopbopaloobop Alopbamboom*, Nik Cohn describes the atmosphere at that time, which was to lead inexorably to the advent and takeover of rock'n'roll:

It's one of the clichéd laws of showbiz that entertainment gets sloppy when times get tough and, what with the depression, the war and its aftermath, times had gotten very tough indeed. Hemmed in by their lives, people needed to cling tight in the dark of dance-halls, to be re-assured, to feel safe again. Reality they could do very well without.

Always, that's the kind of situation that Tin Pan Alley thrives on and songs about moonlight, stardust, roses and bleeding hearts were churned out by the truck-load. The big bands lined up strict and formal in penguin suits, crooners slicked their hair back heavy with grease, the

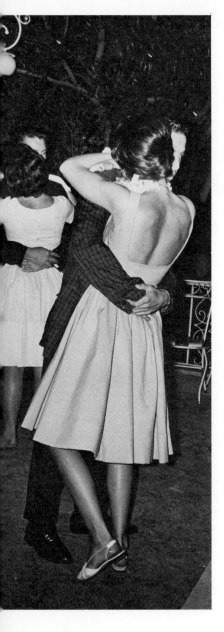

close harmony groups went oo-wah-oo-wah in the background and everybody danced. It was warm and snug like a blanket.

There was no such thing as teenage music then, nothing the kids could possibly identify with.

All this changed in the mid-fifties when a fresh kind of dance music, amalgamating gospel with black rhythm'n'blues and country, began to be promoted on American radio stations. What DJ Alan Freed called rock'n'roll, in order to distinguish it from the unacceptable (because Negro) blues, became an explosive growth industry. Record companies churned out replicas of the new formula and stacked them in juke boxes all over the nation. Spin-off films like *Rock around the Clock* introduced teenagers to the movement vocabulary of rock dancing and television programmes like 'American Bandstand' infiltrated the home and were soon copied abroad. The *New York Times* felt obliged to quote a psychiatrist who declared

When couples actually touched, in the heyday of rock, they tended to dance like these high school kids in California the music to be a communicable disease and a worrying symptom of the growing teenage rebellion.

The TV shows were particularly effective because the 'stars' were ordinary high-school kids with whom any teenager could identify. Young people learned the new styles from watching their peers on the box or, in some instances, following directions incorporated in rock lyrics, like those for the Madison and the

Even pop superstars did not object to appearing on the TV rock shows: here Ringo Starr, in proper Ted gear, dances with an anonymous partner

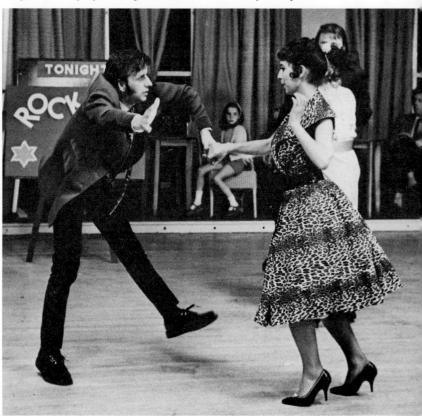

Tennessee Wig Walk. In a song with the latter title, Bonnie Lou belted out instructions which ran something like:

> Put your toes together, knees apart,
> Bend your back and get ready to start,
> Flap your elbows just for luck,
> And you wiggle and you waddle
> Like a baby duck ...

To the uninitiated, the dances looked bewilderingly similar, but teeny-boppers were aware of subtle differences in gesture and floor pattern, and devoured each trend as it surfaced, however momentarily. Within the enclosed teen society awkwardness or inhibition at the weekly 'hop' led to rejection and taunts of, 'He's such a square'. A popular song queried plaintively, 'Do you love me, now that I can dance?'

When Presley introduced the pelvic thrust to the mass media, inciting public hysteria, dance styles became explicitly sexual. During the fifties kids had more money to spend, and the shrieks of parental outrage spurred them on to greater defiance. New uniforms were adopted: in England 'teddy boys' kitted themselves out in drainpipe trousers and long, drape jackets, fluorescent socks and pointed-toe shoes. By the time Elvis was drafted into the army, in 1958, other cult heroes had emerged – actors like Marlon Brando and James Dean, singers like Little Richard, Buddy Holly and Eddie Cochran plus any number of vocal groups, the classiest of which were black.

With the fast, spontaneous turnover of dance fads, teenagers started to separate completely on the floor. Couples might face each other, but seldom touch. Any communication came from a shared appreciation of the beat. The athleticism of jiving, with its back flips and hand springs, gave way to narcissism, and individuals grooved in their own private world. What had been

---

'The King', Elvis Presley, showing what a pelvic thrust is all about, in the film *Jailhouse Rock*

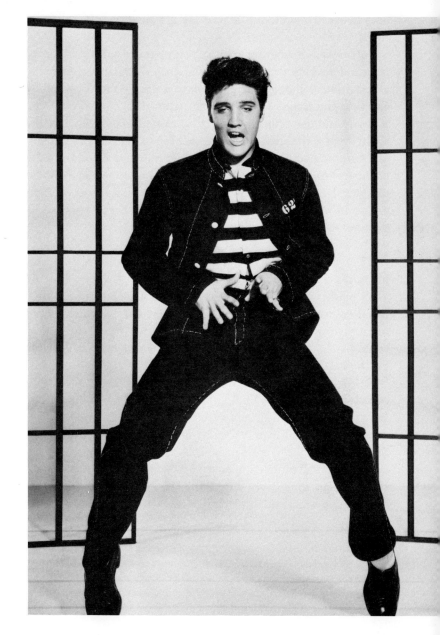

an extroverted imitation of the sex act became a self-centred ritual.

1960 was a downer for rock culture. Record sales were dropping and the kids were getting bored. Frantic businessmen in the entertainment industry latched on to a dreary disc by Chubby Checker and hyped it into an international fashion. The Twist was safe and marvellously easy to do. Anyone could manage the slight bend of the knees, a side-to-side hip swing and a simultaneous pumping action of the arms, while rolling over on the sides of the feet to maintain balance. Predictably, the media deplored this latest example of 'jungle decadence' while dance schools cashed in with snap courses and Chubby Checker lost pounds by demonstrating how to move as if you were 'drying your back with a towel'.

The substitution of the word 'back' for 'bottom' indicates the oddly wholesome image of the Twist. For the first time the adult market picked up on a teenage craze. Discotheques, which had mushroomed during the fifties, advertised Twist bands and the twisting activities of jet-set socialites filled the gossip columns. A social dance style was deemed universally acceptable for the first time in years.

A whole rash of interchangeable dances followed, a few with actual steps: the Hully Gully, the Duck, the Mashed Potato, the Pony, the Frug and dozens of others. Except for the rare line dances, in which the crowd splits into parallel rows to perform the Popeye or the Watusi in unison, the emphasis continued to rest on the individual, and soon the excitement ebbed. Professional go-go girls were hired to dance in clubs, garbed in provocative gear, and slick chorus lines replaced the amateurs

---

(Above) A Limbo queen, Maria Jackson, making clear the connection between black traditional dances and modern pop styles
(Below) Swedish teens practising the Twist in the great out-of-doors. Notice the resemblance to the movement above

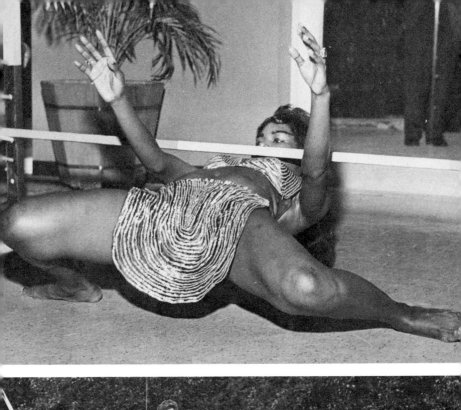

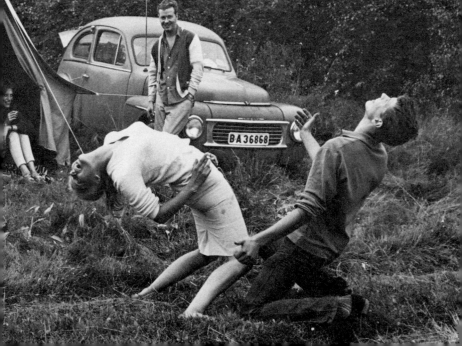

who had once so cheerfully rocked and rolled across television screens.

Meantime, a purer brand of black music, soul, was infiltrating the air waves and was soon taken up by the Mods in Britain. Their opponents, the Rockers (descendants of teddy boys), were fanatically attached to the black-leather/motorcycle culture of the fifties, and they resented what they considered to be an effete obsession with clothes and style on the part of the Mods. The Rockers drank beer and picked fights; the Mods popped amphetamine pills and hung around in West Indian dives, where they danced to modified rhythm'n'blues and Jamaican Ska or Blue Beat. Before long they had their own rock group, the Who, and identified totally with their well-dressed but aggressive act.

The twitching, convulsive Caribbean dances of the day were soon augmented by soul sounds passionately interpreted by superstars like Ray Charles and James Brown, smooth groups on the Tamla Motown label like the Temptations and the Supremes. The majority of the top artists were black American, but by 1963 two English groups had emerged to dominate the world of rock – the Beatles and the Rolling Stones. Pop culture became centred in 'swinging London' and dance styles were developed in Liverpool instead of New York or Detroit. But as the stage shows of the trendiest groups became more elaborate, and the volume of their sound was amplified past the pain threshold by new electronic equipment, teenagers stopped dancing altogether to watch and listen, transfixed.

Certainly there was lots to look at in the rock concerts, even before psychedelia set in. Pete Townshend of the Who would handle his guitar like a machine gun, sometimes bursting into a rage and demolishing it against the speakers. The Beatles would shake their gleaming moptops, every movement provoking screams and fainting fits from their massed fans, while

Teds, resplendent but surly. They jived a lot
(Insert) Rockers, supposed successors to the Teds. They didn't dance. Too busy beating up Mods

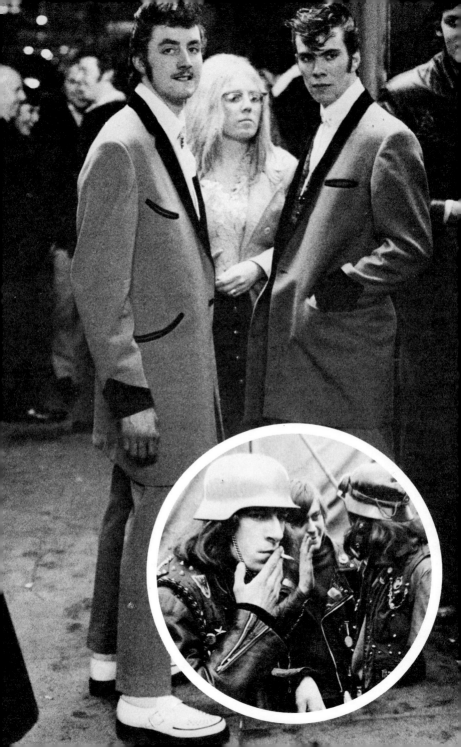

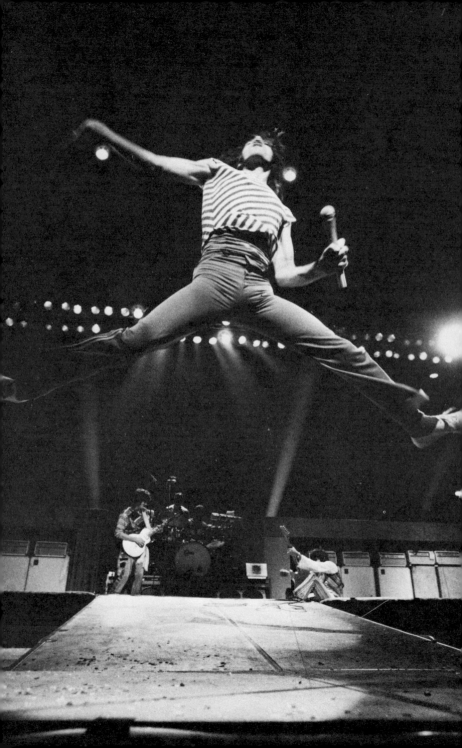

Mick Jagger of the Stones created a performing style all his own, a bizarre mixture of writhing, shuddering effeminacy and belligerence. Nik Cohn remembered one of Jagger's early stage appearances:

He looked like an updated Elvis Presley, skinny legs and all, and he moved like him, so fast and flash he flickered. When he came on out, he went bang . . . he was all sex.

And he was outrageous: he spun himself blind, he smashed himself and he'd turn his back on the audience, jack-knife from the waist so that his arse stuck straight up in the air, and then he'd shake himself, he'd vibrate like a motor, and he'd reach the hand mike through his legs at you, he'd push it right in your face . . .

A hard act to follow. As the beatniks and peaceniks faded into the rearguard of the sixties' revolution, and pills were replaced, first by hash, then LSD, what little disco dancing still went on became increasingly subdued. There was no space for spectacular action in those crowded clubs, anyway, and when the growing underground culture produced hippies, flower power and acid rock, with Bob Dylan as chief spokesman, pop dance had degenerated into the aptly named 'idiot dancing'.

It is difficult to move in a coordinated manner when the mind is addled by drugs and the senses engulfed by flashing lights and sonic crescendo in imitation of an LSD 'trip'. Dylan himself said recently in an interview in *Rolling Stone* magazine that he couldn't dance to any of his songs. Acid rock was loud, free form and improvised, and the dancing which vaguely accompanied it, shapeless. People wandered off and on the dance floor alone, shaking their bells and beads, or ecstatically whirling around like dervishes.

In 1966 *Time* magazine selected as its Man of the Year, 'The man and woman of twenty-five and under', and commented, 'Never have the young been so assertive or so articulate.'

Mick Jagger in one of his more expansive moments. Note aerial development from Elvis's earthbound hip thrust

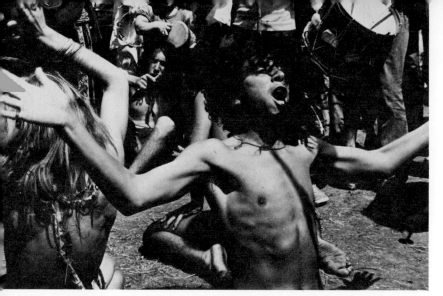

A sixties rock festival featuring a (presumably) stoned youth indulging in idiot dancing

Hippies deserted the psychedelic clubs and flocked instead to huge open-air rock festivals, like those in Monterey and Woodstock. There they serenely lounged around, sometimes breaking into a casual group dance led by a happily stoned individual, or discussing the issues of paramount concern: drugs, sex, the Vietnam war, liberation movements for blacks, gays and women, ecology, the effects of meditation, the New Left.

When this Age of Aquarius faded, pop culture went into a short period of hiatus. Any urge to dance was relieved at a distance by sophisticated rock concerts which evolved into a new form of theatre. Groups like the Pink Floyd and Genesis, soloists like Alice Cooper and David Bowie, employed complex technology and skilled production teams to create spectacular multimedia productions for audiences numbered in the hundreds of thousands. Many of these shows incorporated professional dancers to augment the battery of stage effects – laser beams, split-screen projections, dry ice and inflatables.

But costs skyrocketed and the public became harder to shock

or amuse. Discos returned to favour as the recession of the seventies forced everyone on to a restricted budget. Jamaican reggae had grown in popularity in British clubs, and now it was taken up by fans in America. Reggae has a tight, nervy sound which propels the listener to dance. Frederick Hibbert, one of its originators with his group Toots and the Maytals, instructs:

The idea of the beat is to have the drum casting around, playing off the beat. The bass line goes with it. The rhythm guitar strides on through – one, two, three, four. When you dance, you dance right on the beat. It's a feeling – if you can't feel the beat, you can't do the dance.

A lot of whites fail to follow that beat, so look stiff and out of sync doing reggae movements.

Bob Marley, the biggest name in reggae, who dances even when he doesn't move

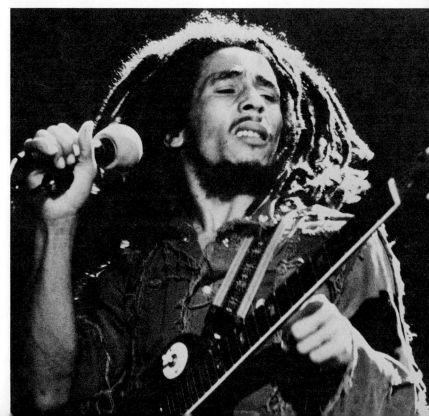

Other minorities have played a key role in the recent resurgence of pop dancing, notably homosexuals who have 'come out' and feel free to mingle socially outside their own clubs, and, in Manhattan, Puerto Ricans who have devised their own Latin sound and dance called Salsa. With new discos opening almost nightly around the globe (rough estimates point to over four hundred in the city of New York alone, some nine thousand in Spain and, unexpectedly, a thriving disco scene in Japan), record companies have rushed to plug 'disco music'. The main variation on the soul formula of the sixties is the length of the records, singles being extended to twelve inches to allow more dancing time per side. The clubs themselves are often based in converted theatres or warehouses which accommodate vast crowds and provide open areas for the most energetic dancing – there are even roller-skating discos in America. Some create fantastic environments, with video screens showing the 'hot' vocalists of the day amidst eye-popping décor. As in Harlem in the thirties, there is a breed of fanatics who take a short nap after they finish work, don their freaky disco gear, dance all night and return to the office, shattered but replete.

In England this phenomenon can best be observed among the survivors of the movement called Northern Soul. Cities such as Wigan, Blackpool and Leeds host modern marathons, to which devotees flock, arrayed in the requisite roomy trousers or sports wear, to do their own frantic version of the Jitterbug to soul music with a pile-driving beat. In gay clubs it seems to be the rule to strip for action, dancers emerging from the gents' loo dressed in boxing shorts and running shoes. Adidas bags are seen in the most unlikely places.

Stylistically, almost every rock style of the past two decades pops up somewhere. At the time of writing the most acceptable

---

A hard-working solo dancer in a gay disco in London. Gentleman in rear stripped for action, wearing shorts and sneakers

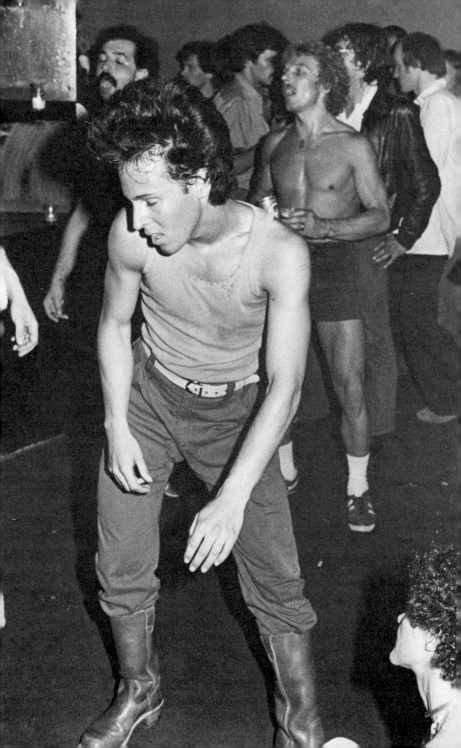

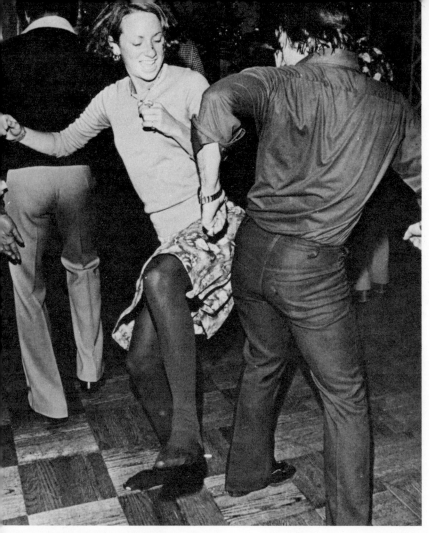

The Bump: a basic form of contemporary disco communication

dances are the Bump, which involves slamming some portion of
the anatomy against a partner and swerving away off the beat, and
different versions of the Hustle which, amazingly, is sometimes
performed in the conventional social dance position. (One disco
mag advised the uninformed to learn this stance by watching

ballroom dance competitions on television.) There is also a group dance known as the L A Hustle, but collective action remains a rarity. Disco dancing of the seventies looks more structured and exhibitionistic than the formless idiot dancing which preceded it, and the footwork can be highly ornate, hence the switch from platform shoes to rubber soles and sneakers. However much the serious followers of rock deride the disco scene, an industry which, according to a speaker at the 1977 Billboard Disco Convention, generated four billion dollars in less than five years, will not easily die out.

The same pop pundits have been prophesying the demise of punk rock almost since it emerged in London, late in 1976. Punk, otherwise known as the new wave or dole queue rock or access music, is based on the nostalgia of today's teens for the excitement of early rock'n'roll, before the rebellion was defused by the media, and the singing stars and supergroups became multinational corporations. Created by adolescents (many of the musicians are only in their mid-teens and boast minimal training) for adolescents, punk is regularly announced as a return to the basics: fast, violent rock performed in clubs small enough to restore the contact between audience and performers lost in the massive rock concerts of recent years. The lyrics, such as they are, seldom refer to sex or love (considered to be old-hat and bourgeois) but rather to unemployment, boredom and aggression. 'Up Yours' is the title of a raucous ditty sung by a group called X-Ray Spex (their soloist is Poly Styrene) while members of the Clash bellow,

> Career opportunities
> The ones that never knock
> Every job they offer you is to keep you out the dock

and Generation X intones,

> Youth youth youth,
> Never wanna be an adult
> Youth youth youth,
> Always wanna be in revolt.

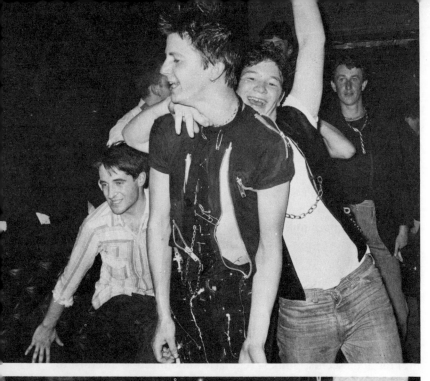

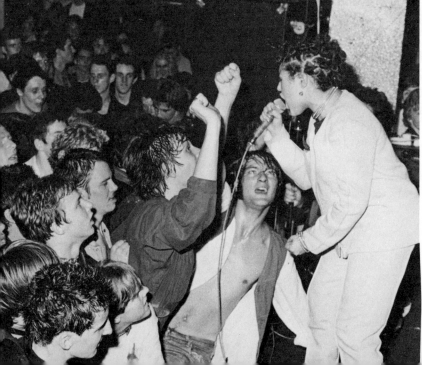

Punk followers festoon themselves with notably eccentric gear, and in consequence are hotly pursued by press photographers risking their ear-drums to invade the congested, steaming clubs. Certainly the spectacle of dozens of punks doing their own anti-dance, the Pogo (also referred to as the Grapple or High Rise Jump), razor blades and safety pins dangling from ears, nostrils and carefully ripped garments, neon-coloured spiky hair jolting up and down in the gloom, is a memorable sight. In the *New Statesman* Mark Kidel described the scene at a 'seedy temple of rock' in Plymouth, in south-west England:

All the punks, who had been solemnly parading about, came alive: they were 'pogo-dancing', a more crazed and aggressive version of flower power's ecstatic 'idiot dance'. As the lights strobed in time to the thumping music, they jumped around anarchically, occasionally bumping into each other and falling over. They hopped around like kangaroos on ECT, their arms seemingly dislocated, waving about in all directions ...

Due to their habit of chaining themselves together, punk dancing often looks more like fighting – and sometimes, in the crush in front of the stage, when bodies are heaved to the top of the pile, individuals retaliate by punching out wildly and a proper brawl ensues, punctuated by beer mugs flying through the air. A Clash member takes it philosophically, 'Most of them kids, they have a good time. They don't feel good unless they go home via the 'ospital ...'

There could hardly be a greater contrast between the calculatedly scruffy punks and the sequined splendour of competition ballroom dancers, who have developed a rabid following all around the globe. As can be seen on televised contests, ballroom devotees remain loyal to the Foxtrot, the Waltz and the Quick-

(Above) Joyful Punks leaping about in the Pogo
(Below) Punks being inspired by singer Poly Styrene – note raised fists, a typical Pogo gesture. The atmosphere, as required, is close and sweaty

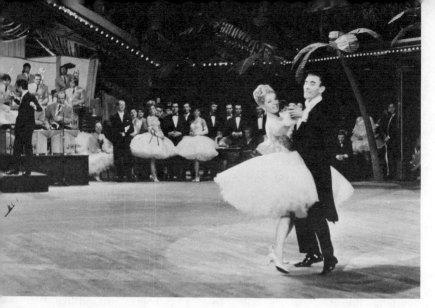

A still from Britain's popular television programme, 'Come Dancing', featuring the elaborate, fluffy gown which too many competition dancers wear, thereby ruining their 'line', i.e. 'the harmonious disposal of the various parts of the body'

step, reserving their flashiest costumes and convolutions for the intricacies of Latin American dances. The first international match was held in 1934, yet these styles seem imperishable: tea-dancing salons can still be found in some cities, in which the regulars sedately trip the afternoon away, and ballroom classes flourish almost everywhere.

Folk-dance clubs have an equally enthusiastic membership these days. Country dances such as Scottish reels, jigs, square dances and the strictly masculine Morris dancing are robustly engaged in by people of all ages.

People who find temporary fulfilment in discos, dance-halls or in folk groups often move on to serious dance training, for the same reason as do the athletes who are discovering the advantages to be derived from studying classical ballet or contemporary dance. More than ever before, this kind of training is freely available.

2 · Training and Participation

Just as rock expanded the popular base of social dance, so the development of modern dance since the turn of this century has inspired a wide variety of people to take up some form of dance training. Dance is now studied by athletes and actors, physicians and psychologists, arts teachers and scholars, as well as by individuals hoping to establish a career in the theatre.

To banish a widely held misconception at once: it is not necessary to be very young nor to possess the physical proportions required by classical ballet to find a niche in the world of professional dance. Those who cannot or do not wish to perform may work as notators or therapists, teachers of theory or technique, administrators or publicists for dance companies. Apart from the stage, the only area virtually barred to those lacking extensive training and experience is choreography; the art and craft of composing dances demands such a high level of skill and original talent that there are less than fifty dancemakers of international standing. But even here there exist new outlets provided by experimental dance, as well as by films and television, night clubs, variety shows and musical comedy. Opera and drama ensembles often employ a resident dance director to arrange the movement element in productions. The more cerebrally inclined can seek a position as researcher or dance librarian; there are also increasing opportunities for writing about dance.

Today dance classes are offered in evening institutes, sports complexes and community centres and are no longer confined to professional training schools and studios. Apart from full-time or regular part-time courses, it is possible to enrol in short, intensive sessions, such as those provided by the renowned summer schools at Jacob's Pillow in the USA and the International Dance Academy of Cologne in Germany, or participate in college seminars open to anyone. It is not possible in a book like this to give specific details of training centres, but useful addresses and reference sources, which should help you to track them down, are listed on p. 183. All I can do here is give a general picture of the opportunities available and the background required for various careers in the field.

Performing

It is a commonplace that the preparation for professional dance is longer and more gruelling than for any other art form or, for that matter, most sports. Classical ballet requires the stiffest apprenticeship because its physical demands are the most artificial involving, for example, ninety-degree turn-out of the legs from the hip and, for women, dancing on the tips of the toes (*sur les pointes* – ballet terminology is in French). In consequence it is difficult, if not impossible, to achieve the right 'line' once a body is fully developed and set in its movement habits.

Enthusiastic parents often choose to enter their offspring in a ballet school when they are barely past the toddler stage. No harm will come of this if the child is allowed to acquire the basics of rhythmic expression and balletic posture gradually. But, unlike modern dance forms, classical technique can cause serious damage to growing bodies if incorrectly taught, and girls forced on point before they are strong enough to cope with the extra strain can end up with bulgy calves and twisted toes. Unfortunately, there is not as yet a universal or even, in the majority of countries, a national licensing system for private teachers, so the only way to ensure that an academy is responsibly run and accredited is to check with dance examining boards for the different training associations.

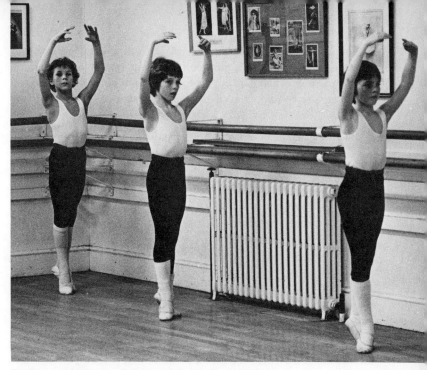

Students of the Lower School of Britain's Royal Ballet

The rigid formality and discipline of classical ballet does not appeal to everyone, and opponents of traditional schooling say it inhibits mental development and individuality. Certainly a concentrated training which lasts at least six or seven years does not allow much time for exploring other areas of life and, as major ballet schools are often residential, young people are caught up in a very insular society.

A rather embittered graduate of the famous Royal Ballet School in Britain recalled the negative aspects of her experience in an interview for a feminist magazine:

> ... you are taught to deny your creativity, intellect and sexuality to conform to an exact, predetermined image. Severe dieting, for example, was common amongst ballet dancers ... in some cases leading to total anorexia. We struggled to conform.

You only have to look at the *corps de ballet* to understand what this narcissistic struggle finally produces: rows of women with identical bodies and expression dancing as swans, nymphs and spirits in perfect harmony, driven and coerced by their ambition to become a 'swan queen'.

Fair comment, perhaps, but this attitude fails to recognize the needs of the art form itself or of those devotees who benefit from immersion in certitudes and find the pursuit of classical perfection deeply satisfying, even addictive.

Girls who aspire to a performing career in ballet should begin regular training by the age of ten, but boys can leave it until later – superstar Rudolf Nureyev did not commence serious study until he was seventeen, and it cannot be said that his achievements have been in any way restricted. A comment in his autobiography gives an insight into the kind of dedication necessary for success in ballet, 'Just as a man consumed by a single passion becomes blind to the rest of the world, so I felt in me the urge, the blind need for dancing and for nothing else.' Auditions are required for entrance into a professional school and scholarships are offered to promising candidates, particularly young men, of whom there is always a shortage except in Russia and other Soviet countries. Age groups are usually defined by the equivalent of the Royal Ballet's Lower (11 to 16) and Upper (over 16) Schools, with entrance examinations held within a year of the prospective pupil reaching that birthday. The curriculum combines academic subjects and theatre arts with, naturally, an overwhelming emphasis on technical dance skills.

After completing the full study schedule, dancers who do not plan to teach (this involves further education) will usually apply for a place in the company to which the school is attached, if any, and failing acceptance will go in for competitive auditions. This is one of the most unpleasant aspects of ballet, for professional rejection can prove shattering to an immature ego.

Once accepted into the ranks of a large ballet company, the rivalry continues, but a career is relatively secure. A female

A *corps* performing a modern work, with Balanchine's New York City Ballet
(Below) A *corps* performing a traditional work, *Giselle*, with the Bolshoi Ballet.
In each case, the necessity for precision is clear. Also, the corporate identity

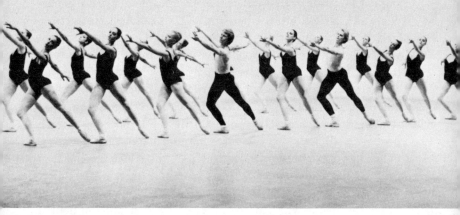

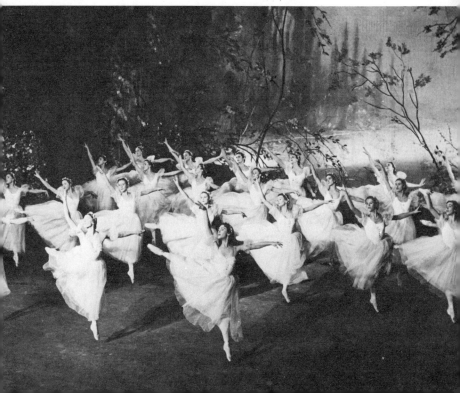

member of the *corps*, the lowest of the low in the hierarchy, would earn at least as much as the average secretary, with the additional perks of world travel, erratic hours (preferred by many to a set routine) and the undeniable glamour of being part of a glittering theatrical establishment. Yearly contracts are standard outside of free-enterprise America, holidays are generous, and salaries for principals and soloists can be high, particularly if they augment their incomes through guest appearances with other ensembles or on television. Many state-subsidized troupes have now introduced early pension and re-training schemes, so injury is less of a hazard, even if the performing life of a dancer remains shorter than that of any other stage artist – seldom extended past the mid-thirties. But nowadays, with people in all walks of life forced by changing circumstances to change jobs, this is no longer as strong a deterrent to a professional dance career as it has been in the recent past.

With regard to social prospects, the popular fantasy of ballerinas being whisked to the altar by rich and influential gentlemen does, in fact, happen quite often, although it must be remembered that there are never more than a few dozen dancers of full ballerina status at any given moment, and most dancers pair off with colleagues, usually those of the same rank within the company.

The image of male dancers as effeminate infuriatingly and unfairly lingers on in western countries. Some of the blame for this misconception lies with the standard costumes – revealing tights in pale colours and brief, elaborately decorated tunics – and more with the partnering convention which, as Royal Ballet star Anthony Dowell says, requires a man to operate 'as a fork-lift truck'. Inevitably, such an enclosed profession can encourage homosexual inclinations, but no statistics prove that there are a higher proportion of gay men in ballet than in any other selected section of the populace. Whatever his private leanings, the male dancer who does not look and move in a virile way on stage will not prosper, unless he is in a drag show.

Of late, charismatic stars like Nureyev and Baryshnikov (both of whom were brought up in a country which glorifies the status of men in dance) have contributed a great deal to a wider acceptance of a career in ballet. The growing involvement of athletes in dance has helped, too. Many a rugged footballer has been shaken to discover just how arduous the normal ballet class is, and an American choreographer found sportsmen queuing up to train with his company after an experiment which involved them in the dancers' daily workout.

The potential benefits of combining certain aspects of athletic and dance training are so great that many countries are now cultivating exchanges, a recent example being the joint sponsorship by the British Arts and Sports Council of a day-long session for weightlifters, gymnasts, runners and dancers. The results of such interaction can be seen in the career of Mary Prestidge, who was a member of both the British Olympic Gymnastic team and, shortly thereafter, the Ballet Rambert. Today she teaches dance in a London sports centre and gymnastics in a dance studio, where her pupils include actors, clowns, dancers and novices in search of interesting exercise.

Mary began her own dual training at the age of five, so finds it difficult to distinguish the superiority of one form over the other. But she does feel gymnasts can learn a lot from dance, particularly in the areas of balance, placement and turns.

Gymnastics is becoming very scientific, very technical, very correct. But the training falls down in developing an awareness of the whole body, the feeling of flow, the sense of balance. Because they're taught to be competitive almost from the beginning, gymnasts don't enjoy movement for its own sake. They may be able to stretch but they can't bend, so they'll do a jump with stiff legs and land so hard they hurt themselves.

Ballet helps gymnasts with line and coordination. Virtually all the girls study it now, but a lot of male coaches think it is frivolous or a waste of time. That attitude is understandable because the competitions for men are run on very strict lines, and there is not so much of the show business element, the 'twiddly' bits, that you find in the women's routines. The posture of some gymnasts, even good ones, can be really bad. No dance company would allow it.

Generally speaking, contemporary dance has more to offer the average participant than gymnastics or ballet, not least because it is possible to commence training at a later age – eighteen and upwards. Modern techniques have evolved from the movement experiments of several high-powered individuals, and this emphasis on personal rather than corporate expression has continued to the present day. The resulting multiplicity of styles means that an enthusiast can sample a wide spectrum of forms before committing himself to a particular school.

America being the birthplace of modern dance (although there were important German pioneers in this field, between the two world wars), the majority of important teachers, studios and companies are based in that dance-mad nation. London boasts an authorized school of Martha Graham technique, the only one outside of her own in Manhattan, and there is a sprinkling of good technical coaches in cultural capitals like Amsterdam, Cologne, Paris, Sydney, Tel Aviv and Toronto. But it is more or less taken for granted that a serious student of contemporary dance will at some point explore the New York scene, which incorporates an extensive studio circuit. Unfortunately, mediocre teachers abound everywhere, and although badly taught modern is not as potentially harmful as badly taught ballet, it is all too easy to waste a lot of time, effort and cash on classes which offer little opportunity for development. You just have to shop around. Private tuition is often offered on a one-off basis, so it is possible to try a single session before signing up for a series or an entire term. A warning: so-called master classes for professional or advanced students given by the top teaching names tend to be packed out, sometimes with pupils of varying levels of accomplishment. For those who do not fancy being crammed into a sea of sweaty bodies, with instruction delivered through a microphone, it is advisable to ask permission to watch. Some

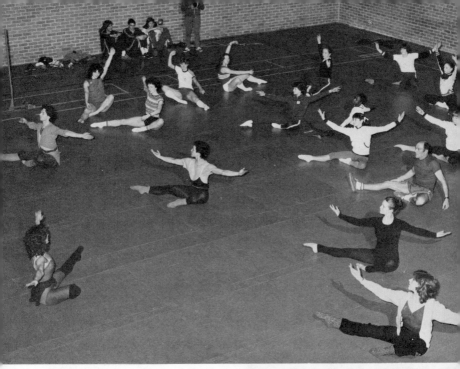

A dancer attempting to teach a motley collection of amateurs and athletes the skills of her particular trade (without notable success, judging from the back rows)

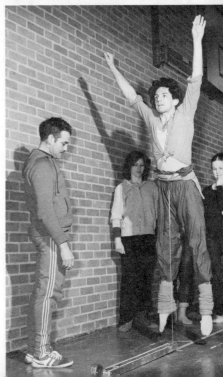

Leigh Warren of the Ballet Rambert being tested for 'explosive leg power' with some watchful athletes, at a combined dance–sports workshop

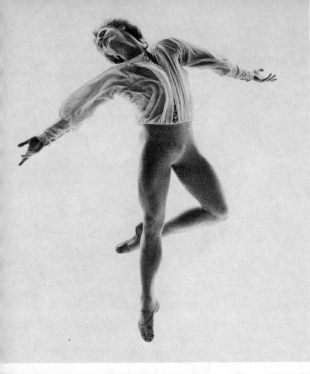

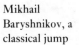

Mikhail
Baryshnikov, a
classical jump

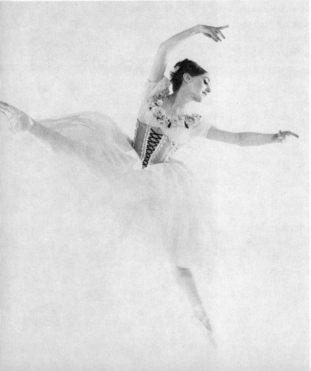

Brenda Last of the
Royal Ballet,
another kind of
classical jump

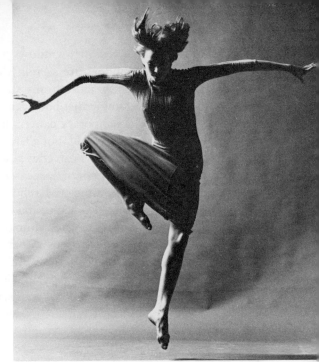

Siobhan Davies, a
funky, modern
jump in a solo
called 'Harmonica
Breakdown', by
Jane Dudley

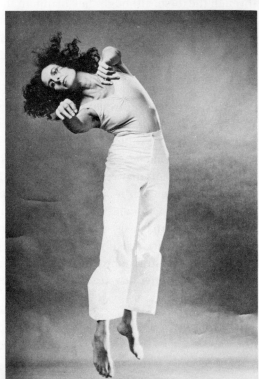

Trisha Brown doing
her very own style
of a contemporary
jump

dance studios provide viewing windows for this purpose.

Because modern techniques are so much more flexible and individualistic than ballet, practically any size or shape of body is acceptable, always assuming that body can meet the demands of a particular style. Contemporary dancers battle to keep their weight down, just as classicists do, but a large frame or unusual proportions need not preclude a career as a performer.

This is not to imply that modern dance is any less taxing than ballet. A daily class is required and rehearsals can be more arduous, for casts are generally smaller and the responsibility of each dancer correspondingly greater. But the movements are based on a natural flow which frees rather than restricts the body, so there should be less stress and fewer accidents. Whereas ballet dancers seek to defy gravity and create the impression of extraordinary lightness, modernists make use of weight and deliberately carve out their own space. There has been considerable interchange of accepted techniques during the past two decades: ballet dancers are now more supple through the torso, although they maintain the importance of the five basic positions of the turned-out feet and related arm movements, while modern dancers may joyously leap and spin, point their bare feet and emulate the speed of their erstwhile rivals.

Partly as a form of insurance, professionals in the more competitive dance centres usually study a range of technical disciplines. Vital differences remain, however, the most obvious being the choice of subject matter or theme. Modernists eschew fairy tales, beaming peasants and dazzling pyrotechnics, and deal with more relevant matters of social or personal concern.

Earning a living in modern dance is a much more perilous business than joining an established ballet troupe. Contemporary ensembles can consist of any number from two up to a maximum of about thirty members, and as very few are subsidized all year round, they function seasonally, filling in performance gaps by means of individual teaching assignments or a corporate residency in a college. Such is the general pattern in Canada and the USA, although accredited modern companies elsewhere can offer annual contracts and the same benefits as those conferred on their wealthier, classical colleagues. Avant-garde experimentalists are forced to fend for themselves, which can mean spending some part of the year subsisting on unemployment payments. In communist countries, with the exception of Cuba, modern dance as westerners know it is not performed.

As well as ballet and contemporary dance theatre there is also the commercial world of dance: musicals, variety shows, night-club acts, television and films. Many 'serious' dancers turn to these outlets during periods of unemployment, while others prefer show-business work because it is less technically demanding and better paid. Good looks are a requisite, or at least the ability to appear attractive in costume, and so is training in jazz and/or tap plus some background in classical or accepted modern styles. An extroverted personality and singing talent helps, too. Jobs are advertised in the trade papers and the main dance studios, and handed out after auditions; competition can be tough. Performers are usually tied to run-of-the-show contracts, which may mean months or even years doing the same role if a show is successful.

Alternative dance careers

The first dance degree was established in 1926 at the University of Wisconsin in America, and since then academic dance courses have mushroomed on campuses throughout the country. The *Dance Magazine Directory* lists hundreds of American institutions offering movement studies, and degrees in pure dance or performing arts including dance can now be obtained at a handful of colleges and universities in Canada and Britain. This number will unquestionably increase over the next few years. Dance was originally allied to the drama or physical education department because of shared facilities, but recently it has become an independent faculty or joined with fine or theatre arts programmes in some schools, an important change in status.

Subjects to be studied for such a degree include a range of dance techniques, composition, dance history and criticism, notation (the most widespread systems are those of Benesh, Eshkol or Laban, although other approaches may be used), anatomy, aesthetics, music, teaching methods, kinesiology (the science of human movement), theatrical production, repertory, improvisation and therapy. A fascinating variety, which accounts for the rapid expansion of the discipline, although there are still huge areas of dance awaiting analysis and documentation.

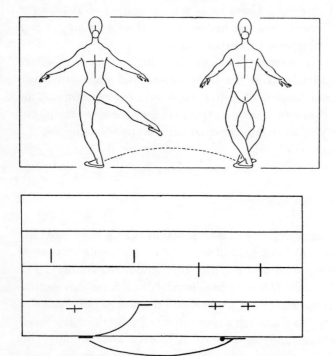

An example of Benesh notation: very easy to analyse, if not to interpret

The American critic Marcia B. Siegel once wrote that 'Dancers are a people without a past.' Fortunately, resource centres for dance research are now being developed, although there are insufficient outlets for the number of scholars. The most comprehensive are the Dance Collection of the New York Public Library, which houses a wealth of visual and sound material as well as written documents, and Stockholm's Dance Museum, with extensive records of Far Eastern dance, as well as other movement forms. The New York Library has issued a twelve-volume catalogue of its dance archives, and runs a world-wide microfilm service. Dance schools and university libraries should at the very least stock the basic literature, and there are theatre collections in many countries which include dance costumes, notation scores, tapes of music and interviews, programmes and films of performances, photos, designs and publicity material.

Students who wish to qualify in a specific area like teaching, notation or therapy should apply to schools which offer concentrated training, rather than tackle a more general degree course. Technique teachers do not need diplomas to work in private schools or professional dance companies, but educational requirements must be satisfied if they want to work within the state system.

This is seldom the case with dance therapy, because it is a relatively new area and practitioners may be drawn from related occupations: psychology, medical massage, chiropractic, osteopathy, physiotherapy or dance education. Some noted therapists have devised their own methods over long years of experience, but lack paper qualifications. Basically, the idea is that both physical and mental ailments can be relieved by involvement in general dance activities, rather than by applying a particular technique. Body awareness is increased by breathing and co-ordination exercises, through improvisation, social and folk dances or encounter sessions. Although therapy is most often practised in hospitals and schools for the handicapped, there is

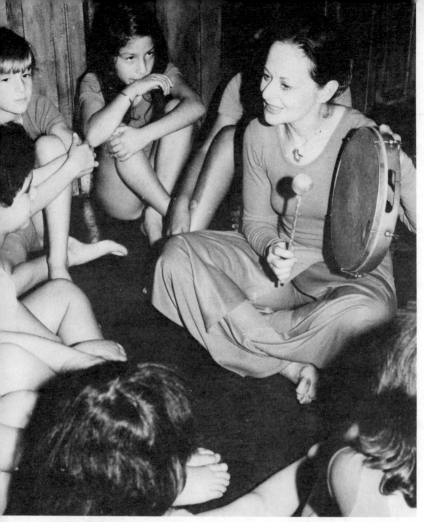

Dance therapist Maria Fux from Argentina, working with deaf children in her school (they can feel vibrations from the tambourine, even if they can't hear them)

also a demand for specialists in movement techniques which help otherwise healthy individuals to understand and overcome physical tensions. Actors and singers, for example, may study body control or the methods developed by Alexander or

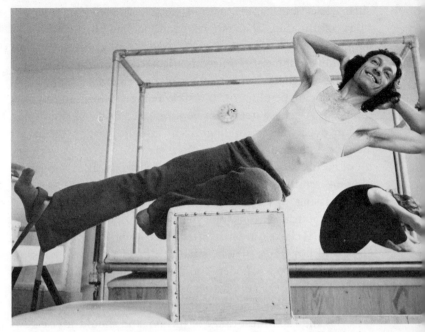

Dreas Reyneke demonstrating a typical exercise on his 'body conditioning' equipment, in London. The spine is straight, albeit at an angle, supported partly by the foot under a noose

Feldenkrais in order to eradicate postural problems, thereby releasing latent energy which helps their artistic activities. Books on the established systems are widely available but in order to teach or administer therapy it is, of course, necessary to study under a recognized authority.

Dance for fun and fitness

Easier access to theatrical and educational dance performances has been accompanied by something of a boom in participation. Nowadays people want to have a go themselves, rather than

53

sitting back and gaping at the spectacle. Dance classes can be more stimulating than sports, and, lacking the element of competition, offer a more creative route to physical well-being. The only equipment required is a leotard and tights, or similar clothing which permits freedom of movement yet shows any faults, and, depending on the style being studied, appropriate footwear. All these items can be purchased at dance boutiques, and in departments for lingerie or athletic gear in the larger stores. Modern dance pupils often wear heavy socks with the toes and heels cut out, to prevent foot cramps. It may seem an obvious reminder, but men must wear a dance belt or risk embarrassing, perhaps painful, exposure.

For practical reasons, the majority of open, as opposed to professional classes, are held after office hours and during weekends, and nowadays may be sited in a great variety of halls. As long as the floor is wooden and the heating adequate, luxuries like large mirrors, a supporting *barre* and changing areas can be dispensed with. Commercial studios usually provide the best facilities and the widest range of tuition, and should advise newcomers on how to choose an introductory course. When in doubt, ask to watch a class, or glean information from the regulars. Teachers advertise in specialist publications or circulate details through education authorities, local arts associations and youth, arts and sports centres.

Modern dance techniques and jazz or tap are more likely to appeal to late starters than classical dance forms, but many people are discovering that oriental disciplines like *t'ai chi chu'an* or *hatha* yoga, which emphasize stillness and proper breathing, can be extremely helpful, particularly for bodies that are tense and/or seriously out of condition. An improvisatory, communal approach to movement is becoming increasingly popular as well, for no technical skills are required, only a willingness to work with others in an exploratory format. These 'natural dance' groups encourage audience participation when they give performances, and members of the public may be astonished to

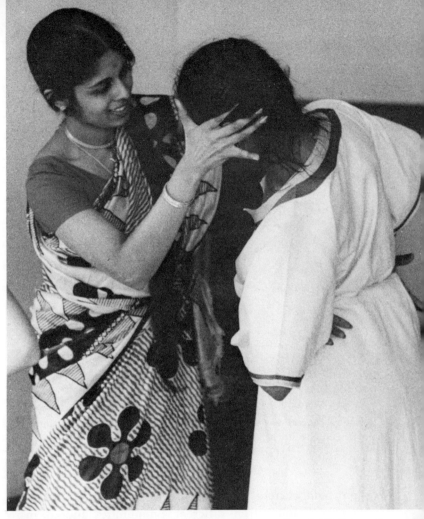

Tara Rajkumar, an Indian Kathakali dancer, teaching eye movements to a London student

discover they are having a wonderful time swaying in a conga line or rolling over total strangers on the floor. Improvised numbers can make effective dance theatre, and instil a satisfying sense of accomplishment.

There is a clear relationship between this dance-for-all philo-

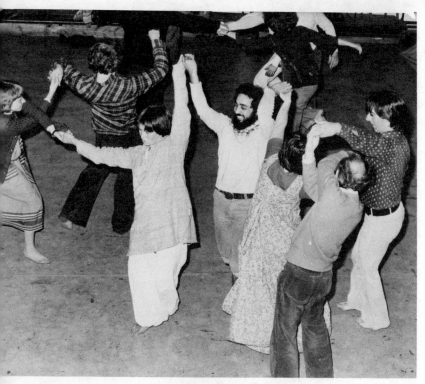

'Natural dancers' having fun at a communal gathering. They probably had not met each other before this event

sophy and current concern with self-help and cooperation among individuals from different communities. Indeed, many groups run weekend and holiday courses in peaceful countryside settings, and give all-day family sessions which generate a casual, friendly atmosphere. Natural dance can be regarded as free-form, contemporary folk dancing, and encourages the same kind of collective rapport.

Somewhat more athletic versions of this non-stylized approach to movement are winning new followers, particularly contact improvisation, which its creator, Steve Paxton, calls 'a conversation on a physical level'. Linked to Eastern techniques is a discipline known as release work, a solitary process during which ideal anatomical images are gradually transferred from the mind to the body.

These and other modern forms, offer everyone the chance to dance.

A Hustle class in a London school devoted to dance for everyone, Dancercise

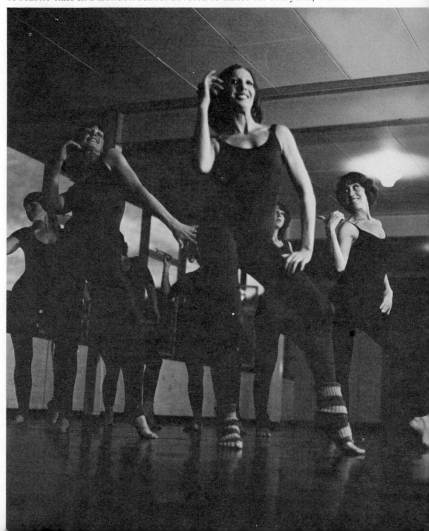

A day in the life of two dance students

PHOTOGRAPHS BY DAVID BUCKLAND

Julie Barnsley and Peter Okun Jones are full-time students at the London School of Contemporary Dance, founded in 1966 to provide teaching in modern techniques based on the work of Martha Graham, and now recognized by the British government as a College of Further Education. It has 120 pupils in the professional training course and over 200 adults, teenagers and children taking part-time classes. Based in a building called The Place, the studios and theatre are also the home of the London Contemporary Dance Theatre.

Both Julie and Peter came late to dance. Julie had studied ballet and tap casually from childhood, but it was not until she saw a performance by the London Contemporary Dance Theatre in her native Yorkshire when she was fifteen, that she decided to try to make a career of dancing. 'For the first time dance meant something to me – it was a whole new movement language,' she says, 'and I felt I had to learn more. Two years later I auditioned at The Place and won a scholarship. I was so excited and happy.'

Peter's first exposure to modern dance came when he was visiting his brother in New York, and was dragged along to see the Alvin Ailey Company. 'I was really into disco dancing and I knew I was good. After seeing Ailey's dancers I went home and tried to do some of the same steps. I couldn't, and I was angry and surprised. By that time I was already almost twenty-five, but I enrolled in ballet classes, and worked with a German "expressive movement" teacher until I had reached a standard where I could apply for full-time training. At my age there wasn't much point in taking more than a one-year course, so that's what I've done, combining the classes with some performing.'

Julie performs too, with a group of senior students who call themselves Junction. She stayed on for an extra, fourth year, in order to polish her technique, teach beginners and gain more stage experience. 'After all this time being totally self-absorbed it feels wonderful to be able to pass something on to other people, in class. I love teaching but I wouldn't consider doing it professionally for many years to come. You should have a lot of solid experience behind you before you start to teach.'

Julie gave up a place in university and Peter dropped out of his degree course in microbiology in order to concentrate on dance. Neither regrets the decision, although they are aware of the insecurity of their chosen profession, the shortage of performing opportunities, the potential necessity of travelling abroad in order to find a position with a recognized company. After graduation, they both hope to continue their training for a few months in New York, which they feel is the centre for modern dance.

Julie says her commitment to contemporary movement is 'almost religious' while Peter, perhaps because of his mixed heritage (his mother is English, his father Nigerian, and he has lived in both countries), feels most comfortable in the areas 'where different styles cross over – I like all kinds of dance, and still go to discos whenever I can. You have to keep in touch.'

(In fact both Julie and Peter found jobs in Germany – Julie with a modern ballet company, Peter with a touring musical comedy production. He was subsequently given a role in the London production of the musical *A Chorus Line*.

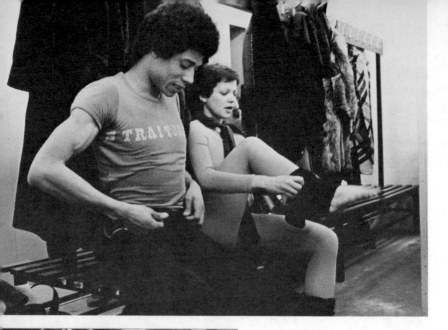

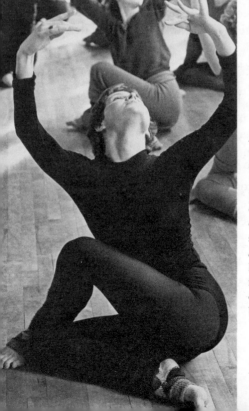

Julie and Peter start every working day in the same manner: changing into dance clothes. The first technique class of the morning begins at 9.30, and as students are expected to have done their own warm-up beforehand, the dressing rooms of the school are usually jammed by 8.30.

Julie in the daily Martha Graham class, which lasts at least an hour and a half. The position shown is one of the standard exercises given during the first part of each session, which concentrates on floor work. This is in contrast to a classical ballet class, which starts with standing exercises at the *barre* to loosen and strengthen the limbs. Graham students sit or lie on the floor, developing the flexibility of the central part of the body and proper breathing.

(Right) Peter being corrected by a body-conditioning expert, during the regular weekly class organized to complement the students' pure technique sessions.

(Below) Julie on one of the specially designed pieces of equipment used only in the body-conditioning studio. This platform, with a movable bar on springs, strengthens the dancer's legs while he or she is lying down, thereby being assured of correct spinal placement. Individual pupils can go to the studio during free periods to work on particular physical problems, under careful supervision.

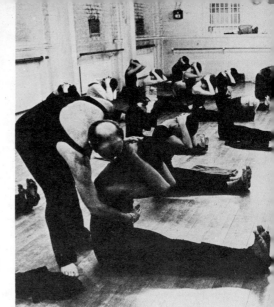

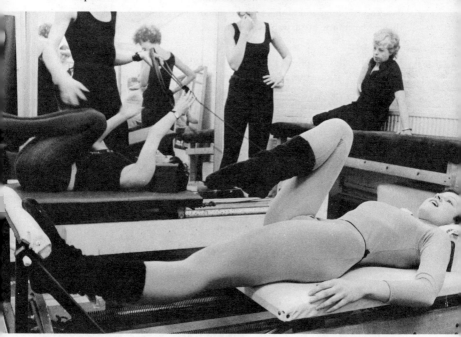

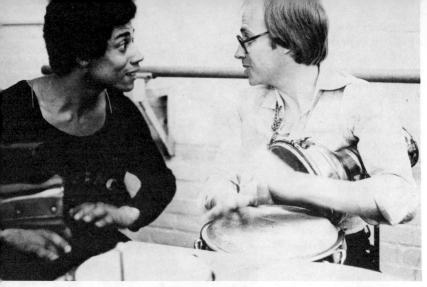

A percussion class, one of several different kinds of musical expression included in the curriculum. Understanding music is a vital part of any dancer's training, and to this end the school offers musical appreciation, theory, harmony, history and voice classes.

Peter and fellow pupils in a lighting class. While some dancers become quite skilled at designing and operating theatre lights, the main concern of these workshops is to demonstrate how stage lighting can influence the look and feel of choreography, and how performers should respond to different lighting situations. The students acquire at least a general knowledge of the lighting board, which operates all the equipment in the school's theatre.

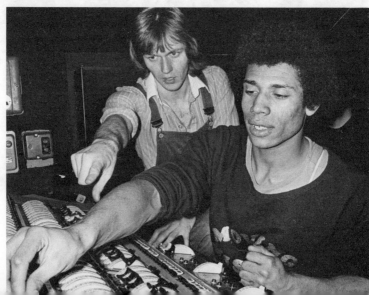

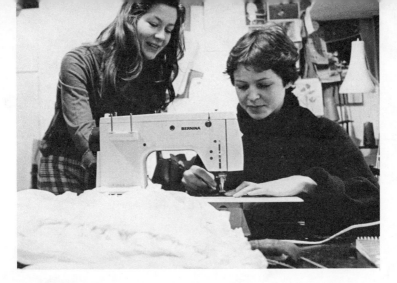

Julie learning to sew a costume, under the guidance of a member of the wardrobe staff. (The male students are given identical training.) Theatre design is part of the stagecraft course which familiarizes the dancers with aspects of the technical presentation of their art form.

Nina Fonaroff, the school's director of choreography, discussing a solo for Julie that has been created by a fellow student. From the first term, all pupils undertake choreographic assignments, and before long see their more successful efforts presented in the theatre to members of the faculty and, by the final year, to members of the public. Guest choreographers teach senior students standard works from the modern repertory. [Photo: Ross McKim]

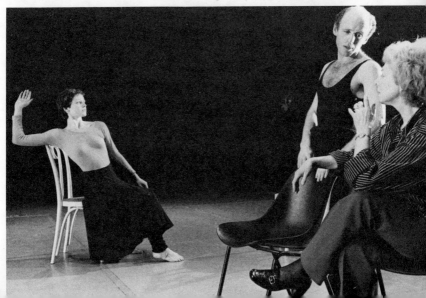

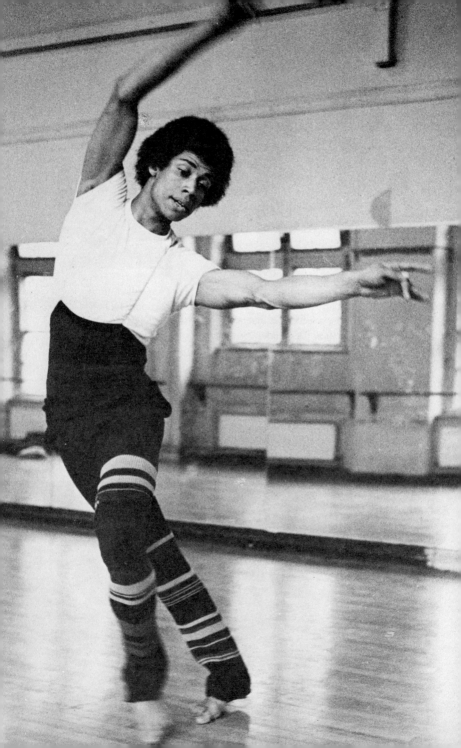

Peter in a jazz class, another movement style in the school timetable. Besides the daily classes in Graham technique and ballet, there are once-a-week classes in jazz and historical and national dance, in order to widen the range of movement expression available to the students.

Now that she is in her final, fourth year at the school, Julie is permitted to teach teenagers introductory dance classes on Saturday mornings. She says, 'I've learned so much from teaching. To give out energy and have it thrown back to you is an amazingly satisfying feeling.'

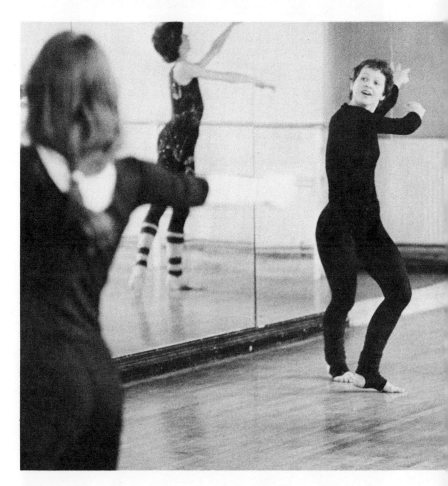

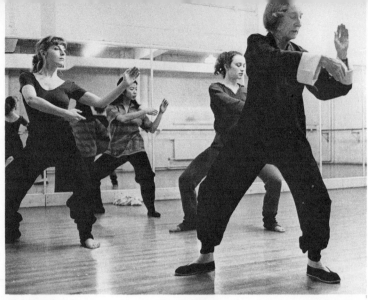

Gerda Geddes giving a class in *t'ai chi chu'an*, an ancient Chinese discipline which introduces students to a different consciousness of their bodies. Based on principles of body–mind harmony, *t'ai chi* can be practised as a martial art form (primarily for self-defence), an active type of meditation or pure dance.

Julie and Peter rehearsing a duet for a school workshop showing.

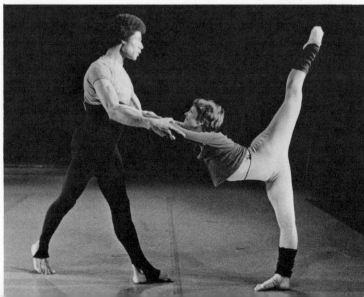

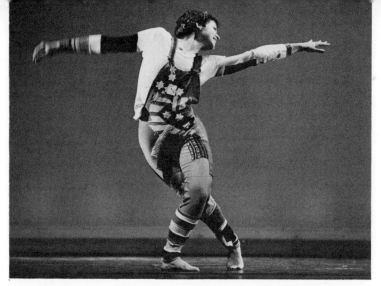

Julie dancing in a London performance by Junction, the contemporary company of which she is a member. Young groups such as Junction generally appear in out-of-the-way theatres and arts centres, augmenting their stage presentations with open classes and lecture-demonstrations to introduce new audiences to modern dance.

Peter as Mephistopheles in a production of *Faust* by the Moving Visions Dance Theatre. Being a full-time student, Peter had to obtain special permission from the school principal before he was able to appear with this small professional company. The income derived from such work is minimal, but the performing experience is invaluable for young dancers.

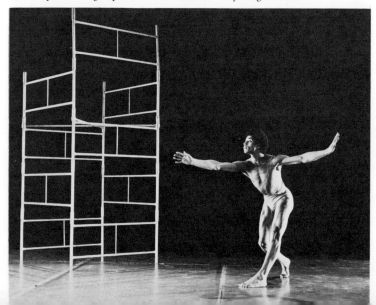

3 · Modern Dance:
Pioneers and Popularizers

My art is just an effort to express the truth of my being in gesture and movement. It has taken me long years to find even one absolutely true movement.

A dancer must listen to his body and pay honour to it. Behind the movement lies this terrible, driving passion, this necessity. I won't settle for anything less.

The first of these quotations comes from Isadora Duncan's autobiography, written shortly before her tragic death in 1927; the second is from an interview with Martha Graham in 1976. Their comments indicate vital similarities between these two great revolutionaries of the dance – an abiding conviction that their art form must involve a searching analysis and representation of human experience, and that movement must spring from within.

Unlike Graham, Duncan did not codify a detailed technique, although she founded schools in a rather helter-skelter way. Her prime importance rests with rhapsodic solo performances and their influences on artists of the time and those who were to follow. But although she was an intuitive genius at improvising movement, she carefully studied the principles of dance. Duncan decided that the solar plexus was 'the central spring of all move-ment, the crater of motor power' and that the pull of gravity shaped every step or gesture. The artificiality of classical ballet would have to be rejected and the feet bared, in order to feel and follow the rhythms of nature better. Stage décor and costume must be simple, so as not to distract from the beauty of the choreography. Such concepts sparked off upheavals in the dance world that have continued to the present day.

Other important pioneers of modern dance were contemporaries of Duncan. Loie Fuller brilliantly manipulated lights and flowing garments to transform herself, as if by magic, into the very essence of a flame, a flower or a butterfly. Ruth St Denis was inspired by a cigarette advertisement featuring an Egyptian goddess to explore oriental dances and themes, translating them into a highly theatrical western idiom. With her husband, Ted Shawn, she co-founded the famous Denishawn School, which taught virtually every movement technique, and a company, to introduce serious modern dance to audiences around the world. After the partnership was dissolved, Shawn went on to direct an all-male ensemble, thereby helping to break down prejudice against dance as a masculine pursuit.

All these innovators were American, and their originality reflected the society that had bred them. Each was to make a singular contribution to the development of a new art form, a new freedom of expression, but it was Martha Graham who became Duncan's heiress apparent. Separately, over several decades, the two arch-rebels expanded the range of dance and gave it intellectual respectability. Their discoveries have changed our perceptions of the human body.

The achievements of both have been documented in currently available books, and Duncan's turbulent life and loves were the subject of a television portrait by Ken Russell (for the British Broadcasting Corporation) and a feature film starring Vanessa Redgrave. Graham, of course, is still very much a force to be reckoned with. Now well into her eighties, she continues to guide her company and to choreograph. She has written incisive essays about her art and her notebooks have been published. Short films record a handful of her major works and in one, *A Dancer's World* (1957), Graham herself discusses the classroom technique on which her achievement is based.

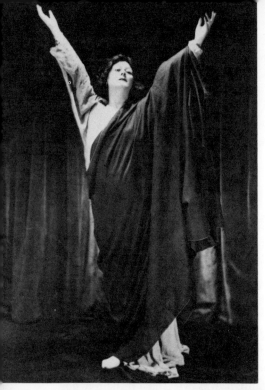

Isadora Duncan dressed in the flowing draperies of which she was so fond. Her bulky appearance would indicate that this photo was taken near the end of her life (circa 1920?)

Loie Fuller in her famous *Fire Dance* (1910)

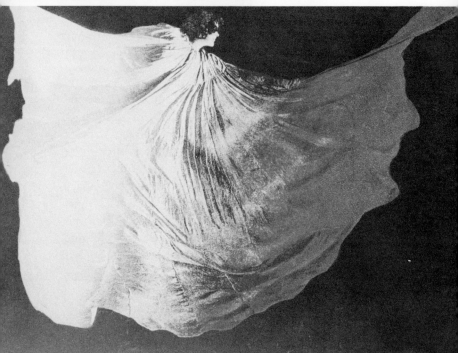

Ruth St Denis demonstrating
the strong oriental influence on
her work in a dance from
The Temple (1908)

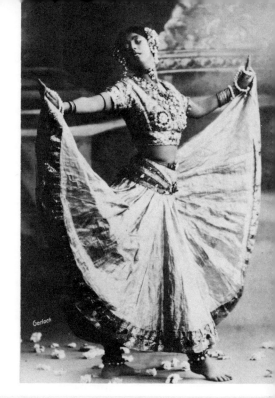

A recent revival of Ted
Shawn's all-male *Kinetic
Molpai*, by the Alvin Ailey
American Dance Theatre
(premiered in 1935)

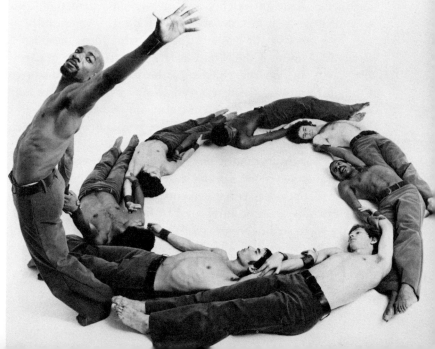

'Movement never lies', declared Graham, and since her solo début over fifty years ago she has indefatigably sought new ways to interpret this principle. Whereas Duncan shocked her public by appearing almost naked, garbed in a flimsy Greek tunic, Graham designed stark costumes which covered the body yet clung to its shape. Duncan kept the performing area empty, except for blue curtains, to contrast with the lavish décor common in the theatres of her era, while Graham collaborated with sculptor-designer Isamu Noguchi from 1934, often incorporating his dramatic, free-standing constructions into the movement. Duncan improvised to the music of renowned composers, Graham began to commission scores written specially for dance. What they shared, however, was the ability to find visual and kinetic images which are startling in their simplicity, yet implacably theatrical. Their ideas on stage presentation have affected not only dance theatre, but the entire spectrum of the performing arts. Over many years Graham evolved a rigorous style of movement which in time expanded into a vocabulary as sophisticated as that of classical ballet. It was a means to her chosen end, the 'affirmation of life through movement', usually channelled through weighty and mythic subject matter – the legends of ancient Greece, aspects of the early American heritage, the inner life of heroines such as Saint Joan, the poetess Emily Dickinson or the Brontë sisters. Her treatment of narrative can verge on the cinematic: the time-scale is distorted through the use of flashbacks and glimpses of the future, and different dancers may represent contrasting aspects of the same individual. Always, whether the dance is narrative or abstract, the movement is there to reveal the emotion.

The Graham method is now the backbone of contemporary dance training everywhere, and she has recently produced video tapes to set out the essential elements. She insists that teachers of the Graham system be authorized by her Center in New York. 'I have spent so much time, sweat and blood on my technique,' she said to the author, 'that I cannot now sit back and allow it

Martha Graham in her 1935
work *Imperial Gesture*,
wearing a costume of her own
design

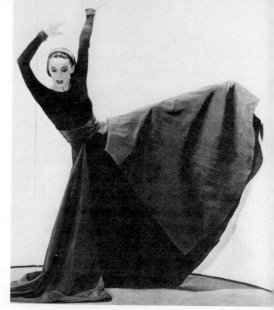

Martha Graham today,
receiving congratulations and
flowers from Mrs Betty Ford,
wife of the former President of
the USA

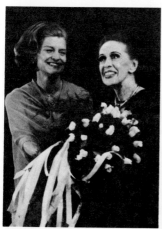

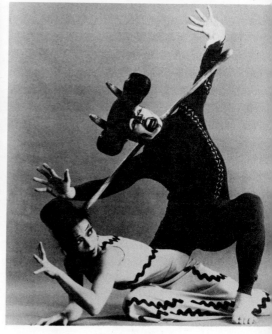

Yuriko Kimura and Tim
Wengerd in the current revival of
Graham's *Errand into the Maze*,
dating originally from 1947

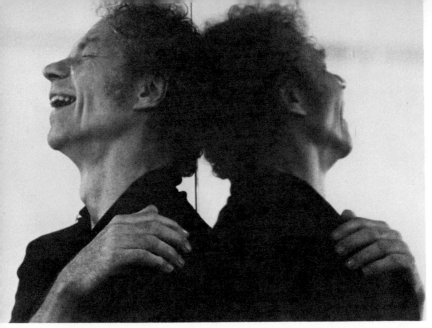

A delightful portrait of Merce Cunningham, taken in 1973

Cunningham's company performing his *Squaregame*. The master peers over the top of the sacks in the background

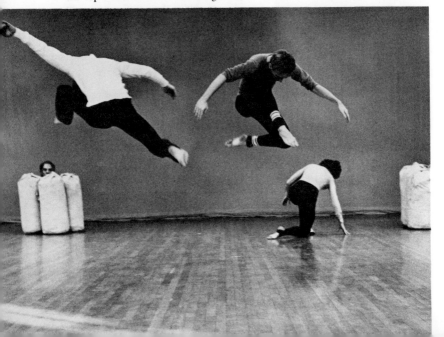

to degenerate in the hands of others, to become two-dimensional or superficial, to focus on stunts.'

Graham has survived public repudiation and personal hardship to receive the highest honours of her country and universal esteem. Her most influential contemporary, Doris Humphrey, another graduate of the Denishawn group, died in 1958 and is chiefly remembered for her testament *The Art of Making Dances*. Humphrey thought of dance as 'the arc between two deaths' and her theories about fall and recovery, balance and imbalance, paralleled Graham's in the establishment of modern dance methodology. She was an impressive performer, and in later life choreographed eloquent works for her protégé, the late Mexican dancer, José Limón. Some of these can still be seen in revivals, but Humphrey's relative obscurity is a reminder of the fickleness of artistic fashion.

In a reversal of the cliché, behind most of these great women stood a man. For a short, significant period Isadora Duncan was involved with the revolutionary theatre designer, Gordon Craig; Ted Shawn organized the framework for his wife's art and attracted athletic young men to their company; Martha Graham's artistic mentor, Louis Horst, encouraged her to seek out native music and had a lasting impact on the modern dance scene through his teaching and writing on dance composition; Doris Humphrey worked with Charles Weidman for almost twenty years, and together they formed a company and a school. The one entirely independent male force of the pioneering generation was Lester Horton. His was the first troupe to employ dancers of every race, and his academy in Los Angeles produced some exceptional pupils who have disseminated Horton's concepts throughout America. Yet it was the feminists who created blazingly potent roles for men, and gave the male dancer an exciting new image.

The leader of the revolt against the female ascendancy in modern dance was Merce Cunningham, a soloist with Graham's company, who broke away to challenge the accepted assumptions of the founders. For more than twenty years he has been the great guru of the avant-garde. An exponent of 'cool' dance, Cunningham said in a *New Yorker* interview, 'I don't even want a dancer to start thinking that a movement means something. That was what I really didn't like about working with Martha Graham – the idea that was always being given to you that a particular movement meant something.'

From the very beginning of his choreographic career, Cunningham has been associated with the composer John Cage, as well as leading painters and sculptors, yet he asserts the separation of the art forms. The movement, sound scores and décor of his creations co-exist, often coming together only in a final rehearsal or the performance itself. For Cunningham, dance is about dance. He never uses a story-line and is completely detached from characterization. Sometimes he determines the sequence of a work by chance, and will toss a coin to decide who is doing what and when. There is no central focus in his use of space: the dancers employ the entire stage area so that the work can be viewed from almost any angle. In fact, Cunningham prefers to present his choreography in something other than a conventional theatre, and seat the audience on three or four sides. Recently he has concentrated on experimenting with video and directing a series called 'Events', in which excerpts from his extensive repertory are recreated to suit a particular setting, like his own studio in New York.

In one main respect Cunningham has imitated the progenitors of American modern dance. He leads a company that bears his name and performs only his works. Like Graham, Cunningham is very much in command, even though his skilled ensemble of soloists may be involved in the creative process. His style looks unique, combining an emphasis on verticality and almost balletic elegance of line with driving energy and natural gestures. Cunningham dancers will throw off a dazzlingly complex sequence of steps and then break to cough, change clothes, ride a bike or do handstands – a far cry from the taut con-

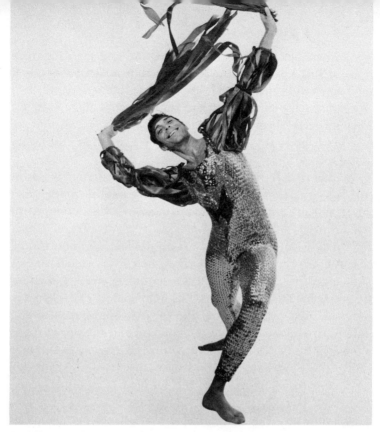

Paul Taylor, who has now retired from performing, dancing his athletic, typically ebullient solo from *Book of Beasts*

trol and spiralling movements typical of Graham's technique.

Cunningham's school and performing unit has been a significant breeding ground for choreographers. Of the many outstanding Cunningham alumni, Paul Taylor is perhaps the most accessible pure dancemaker. This was not always the case. He launched his independence in 1957 with a programme so obscure that it was reviewed by a blank space in the leading dance journal of the day. By the time he assembled his own group, some four years later, he must have acquired what he needed from experimentation for he set about choreographing works that stimulate, but seldom shock. Taylor anticipated the exchanges between classical and modern methods that are now taken for granted, and borrowed from any style that suited his immediate purpose. His genial sense of humour and showmanship allow even his most intricate themes to be readily communicated, and he switches happily from dramatic narrative, to satire and lovely lyrical pieces.

Another widely popular and influential modernist is Alwin Nikolais. 'Nik', as he is known within professional circles, is the closest thing to a wizard working in dance. He has developed an extraordinary type of mixed-media dance theatre, in which movement is only one, albeit a major, element. Not only did he invent a new, technological format, he carried it out single-handed, writing and recording the electronic scores and devising the astonishing lighting effects. His weird gallery of costumes is designed, on occasion, to alter the apparent shape of the body, and his particular dance style is composed of many small articulations, with a twitch in one limb setting off a quiver in another. Unlike the choreographers previously discussed, Nikolais has never enjoyed being on stage, and for long years his principal interpreter was Murray Louis. Louis now heads his own successful company, but the two co-direct a dance foundation in New York and collaborate on the production of dance films. Through these films and their fascinating television programmes, thousands of people in different countries have been able to experience their inventive, witty brand of movement theatre.

Martha Graham echoed the concerns of her era – the discoveries of psychologists, the socio-political upheavals which led to the world wars – while Cunningham, Taylor and Nikolais are just as intensely of their time, analysing the fragmentation of our society and the inroads made by technology on art and nature. Nikolais put this point of view most succinctly when he wrote, 'We must give up navel contemplations long enough to take our place in space.' These innovators have, by virtue of extensive

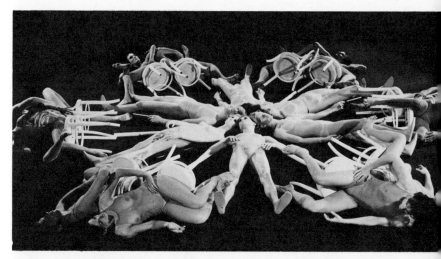

Members of the Nikolais Dance Theatre in action for the television camera (above) and on stage in *Sanctum*

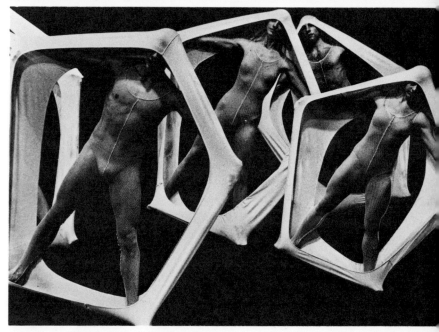

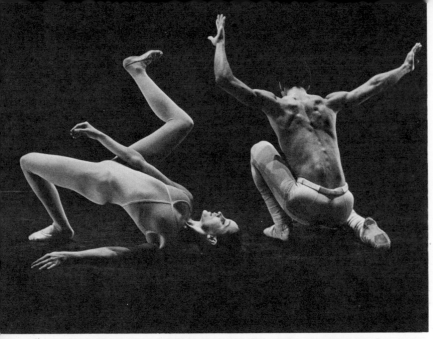

A duet from *November Steps* by Jiri Kylian, the current director of the Nederlands Dans Theater

The same company's production of *Caterpillar* by Louis Falco, showing William Katz's exciting set. The Dutch troupe is noted for the high standard of its designs

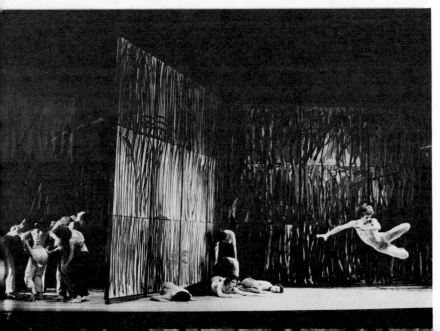

touring, spread their awareness to most parts of the globe. The fact that such travels are regularly subsidized by the US State Department is an indication of the massive acceptance of what was so recently considered to be a daunting art form, and of the pride taken by Americans in their indigenous dance.

The situation of modern dance in Europe is quite different, primarily because it is a mere fledgling when compared with the long established classical ballet. The first Continental excursions into what was then called 'expressive dance' were made by Germans like Kurt Jooss, Rudolf Laban and Mary Wigman, back in the twenties. Nazi persecution forced the disbanding of their centres, and a student of Wigman's named Hanya Holm went to America, there to become a significant force in the new dance, while Jooss fled to Britain, taking his company with him. But few opportunities remained for experimentation during the war years and it was not until 1959, when some Dutch dancers and choreographers left the main ballet company to found the Nederlands Dans Theater, that contemporary movement styles gained a sure foothold.

Teachers of modern dance were scarce, so from its inception the members of the Nederlands group studied and combined classical and Graham-influenced techniques. This practice has since been emulated throughout Europe, as has the Dutch policy of continuous creativity, which may result in ten or twelve premières each year. In contrast to the standard American system, Continental companies draw on the services of many different choreographers, although the director is normally expected to mount a new production when his or her other responsibilities permit. The result has been a blurring of demarcation lines between the traditional categories of dance, though the best ensembles have acquired a distinctive identity of their own.

Britain's oldest professional dance troupe, the Ballet Rambert, was not immune to the goings on across the Channel nor oblivious to the importance of the work displayed by American

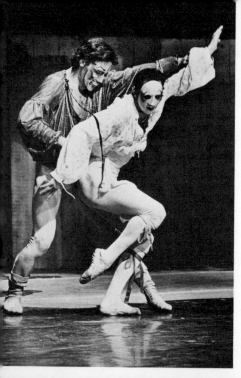

Masked dancers from the Ballet Rambert in its successful, full-length production called *Cruel Garden*

A scene from *Forest* by Robert Cohan, for his company, the London Contemporary Dance Theatre (Anca Frankenhauser and Patrick Harding-Imer are the performers)

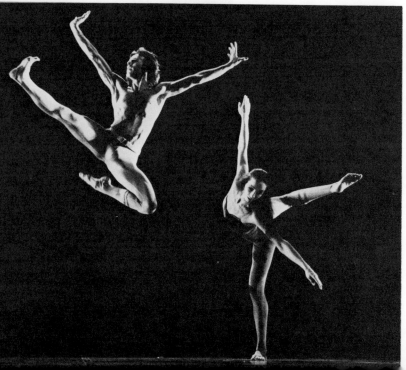

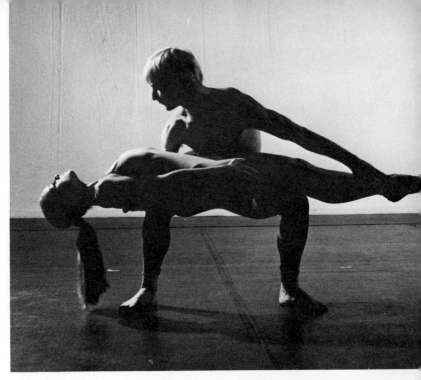

Birgit Cullberg's *Adam and Eve*, danced by her brilliant son, Niklas Ek, and Mona Elgh, in Sweden

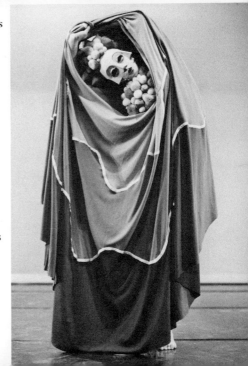

Another masked figure, this time interpreting Domy Reiter-Soffer's work *Journey* for the Bat-Dor Company of Israel

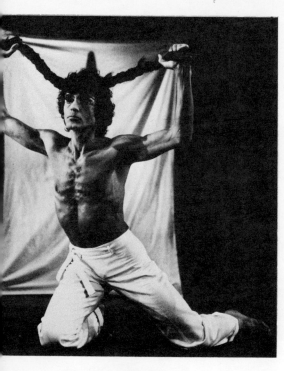

Robert Cohan during his dancing days in Martha Graham's *El Penitente*

(Right) Robert Cohan as teacher, directing students in an English college

modernists on their flying visits. In 1966 the Rambert dropped its classics, and dispersed the *corps de ballet*, retaining only a select band of soloists who were motivated to develop a new repertory with a modern bias. Shortly afterwards Birgit Cullberg set up her own ensemble in Stockholm; by the early seventies there were flourishing contemporary groups in Belgium, France, Denmark, Germany and Portugal. Farther afield, Israel acquired a Graham-based company, the Bathsheva, and its founder, Bathsheva de Rothschild, subsequently formed the Bat-Dor, which uses both ballet and modern styles. These organizations receive a very high proportion of their funds from the government, and are thus able to provide more security for employees than those operating within the competitive, free-wheeling American circuit.

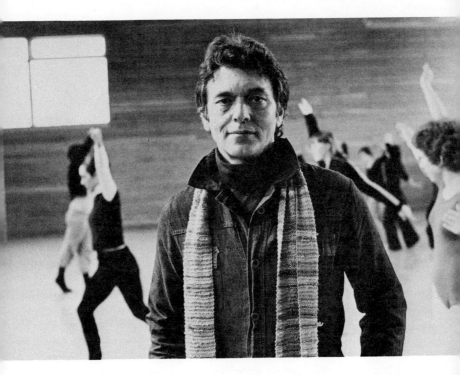

Like the Bathsheva, the London Contemporary Dance Theatre was created by a devoted admirer of Martha Graham. An English hotelier named Robin Howard was so overwhelmed by his first exposure to Graham's company that he arranged its second visit to the UK and opened a trust to subsidize the exchange of teachers and students between her studio in New York and a new school in London. Robert Cohan, a long-standing partner of Graham, was imported to supervise the classes, and by 1969 there were sufficient dancers of a high standard to present a proper season. The public response was enthusiastic and inquiries poured in from young people wanting to learn the Graham technique. In a remarkably short time the transplant had taken, as proved by the company's acclaimed début in the USA during the summer of 1977.

85

Graham believes that national characteristics influence the evolution of a dance form. Geography, social, cultural and religious traditions all colour the way in which people express themselves in movement, although basic principles are universal.

Robert Cohan describes some differences:

As an American, the first thing I noticed about British dancers was their intellectual response to movement. In countries like Israel, the USA, Australia and South Africa, the approach is much more athletic. People spend a lot of time outdoors, and play sports in clothing that exposes the body. Northern Europeans tend to be more introverted – more covered up in every sense.

Now I've learned that in order to teach effectively in, say, England or France, I must explain the exercises verbally, rather than physically demonstrate them. Once students grasp the mental concept they feel emboldened to try the movement, whereas American dancers generally prefer to get on with it, sweat hard and leave a class feeling exhausted.

That's why the Graham style looks different on my company, but it is more a philosophical than a physical reaction. It's important to remember that even in the greatest days of the Graham company we dancers only met regularly for a few weeks at a stretch, just before we began a tour or when we were learning new works. With the European subsidy system companies take class together every day, and there is time to try out movement sequences that will help a choreographer to find what he or she needs. A communal rather than an individualistic approach develops, and this group commitment shows in performance.

The transatlantic modern dance traffic, originally almost all one way, is becoming more balanced, to the benefit of everyone concerned. American choreographers like Cohan, John Neumeier and Glen Tetley have consolidated their reputations in Europe, and commissions from European companies sometimes lead to the invitee returning for a tour with his or her own company. Carolyn Carlson, once a leading dancer with Alwin Nikolais, now runs her own experimental group within the venerable walls of the Paris Opéra. On the other hand, Dutch creators Rudi van Dantzig and Hans van Manen have become

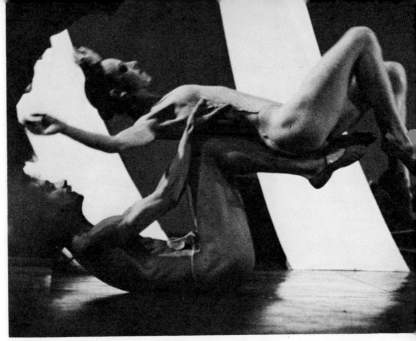

Tip, a work by the young director of the Dance Company (NSW), which is based in Sydney, Australia (the choreographer is supporting Janet Vernon)

familiar names to North American dance fans; a former colleague of theirs, Jaap Flier, gave an enormous boost to the development of contemporary dance in Australia. British dancemakers Norman Morrice and Christopher Bruce have created works for the Tel Aviv moderns, and the young Israeli choreographer Domy Reiter-Soffer commutes between England, Ireland and the USA. And so the cross-fertilization continues, with subtle variations beginning to surface as tastes develop and confidence grows. Europeans, for example, tend to prefer full-length works because of their classical conditioning, so several contemporary companies have responded with works that last for an entire evening. Martha Graham, ever the forerunner, created such a piece, *Clytemnestra*, in 1958, but as Americans are more accustomed to mixed bills, only Paul Taylor has followed her example with any solid success.

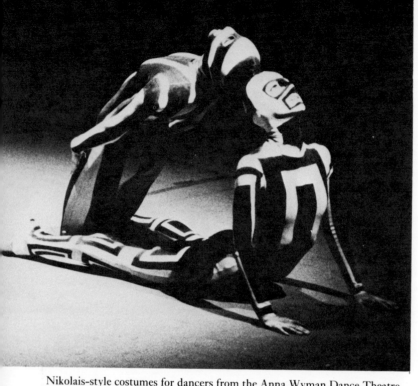

Nikolais-style costumes for dancers from the Anna Wyman Dance Theatre of Vancouver, Canada

Australia and Canada have also entered the modern arena, and their lively new groups are set to make an international reputation, backed by a fast growing public. There are few nations that do not harbour at least one teacher of contemporary technique, and where a good teacher exists, a school and company may soon follow. Far from being a difficult and elusive art form, modern dance has come to be considered, particularly by young people, as a type of theatre with which they can immediately identify. It can illuminate as well as entertain, and a powerful performance will generate an empathy between dancers and spectators that is almost impossible to achieve through other means of creative expression. You do not just feel the movement 'in your bones', but in your muscles, joints, and tingling nerve ends.

Making a ballet

PHOTOGRAPHS BY MALCOLM HOARE

The process of creating a dance work is almost as mysterious to the people involved as it is to the layman. 'Intuition' is the word that crops up again and again in any discussion of the art of choreography. But there are some immediate, practical requirements: dancers, a rehearsal studio, time and, usually, music, played live or on tape. A notator should sit in on every session to record the movements and, if a company has the resources, a video camera will preserve the final result. The costume and/or set designer and the lighting expert participate in the later stages. If the score has been commissioned, the composer will probably have completed his or her work before the first meeting of cast and choreographer.

Sources of inspiration are almost as varied as the choreographers themselves, and intensely personal. This is one reason why dancemakers hate to write programme notes suggesting an interpretation for a work. It is difficult to verbalize the feeling or idea that resulted in a ballet, and choreographers prefer members of the public to respond individually and discover their own meaning. Nowadays few dances have an actual story-line or narrative. The combination of music, movement and design should say it all.

Choreography is a slow, painstaking business and expensive, because actual bodies are the materials from which the ballet is developed. Dancers can be grumpy, injured, hate the music or just feel apathetic about what the choreographer is trying to do. He or she does not only have to be an artist, but a diplomat as well.

89

All this may sound hopelessly vague; so perhaps it would be useful to look at how one particular work got on to the stage. A good example is *Praeludium*, which was first performed early in 1978, in London, by the Ballet Rambert. Glen Tetley arrived from New York to mount the work just before Christmas 1977. The dancers rehearsed daily for six weeks and the result, *Praeludium*, a thirty-minute piece, was greeted with enthusiasm by press and public alike. It is a flowing, romantic ballet, built around the central figure of a woman, played by Lucy Burge. Her partner, the Rambert's associate director Christopher Bruce, makes his entrance quite far on in the work. The remainder of the cast consists of three couples. Tetley asked his long-time collaborators, scenic designer Nadine Baylis and lighting specialist John B. Read, to take responsibility for the visual aspects of the new production. The music is from string quartets composed by Anton von Webern in 1905.

'I discovered the score last summer, and was immediately struck by its transparent youth and purity,' Tetley explained at an orchestral run-through for *Praeludium*.

I find it impossible to even start on a piece unless I am inspired by the music. Once into rehearsals, however, I am equally inspired by the dancers with whom I am working. Lucy, for example, has a wonderfully feminine strength which I've tried to draw on. Having just completed a work about unrequited love for American Ballet Theatre, I wanted to make something serene and centred for the Rambert. Lucy has that very special quality of stillness. So those were the components of *Praeludium*: the score, the individual dancers, and the mood I was in at that time. I've learned not to plan anything in a cerebral way, but to respond to every new influence of the moment. To choreograph is to discover.

Designer Nadine Baylis explained her contribution:

Once I had talked to Glen and watched rehearsals I began to think of visual means that would bring out the kind of movement he was using and reinforce his ideas. In *Praeludium* the movements seem to come from the earth, the dancers' limbs curl and intertwine, so I decided on a sparse set made of curved, twisted steel tubes which would resemble stylized trees.

I always listen to the score when I am doing my designs, so the colour of the costumes, particularly the orangey-red dress for Lucy, were inspired by the paintings and woodcuts of the music's period – the turn of the century. I dyed the fabrics myself and changed Christopher's costume from green to brown to a dark bordeaux red before I was satisfied. There was no time for working drawings, only a model for the set, so I was very reliant on the contribution of the metalworkers and my marvellous costume-maker.

Lighting designer John B. Read's involvement was not quite so time-consuming, but he had his own challenges to meet.

Tetley's works are more complex to light than those of other choreographers because there are certain sections that require very delicate handling, in terms of light and shade. I watched three run-throughs this time (normally I get by with only two) and made notes on anything that popped into my mind – the feelings I had about the work. Only then did I begin to think about the design.

Nadine and I work together very closely. We concentrate on trying to emphasize the dancers in the space. It's not necessary for me to tell her exactly what I plan to do, but I let her know what area of colour we'll be using. Her sets are so good that they light themselves, and she is unselfish enough to allow me to include my own interpretation of the ballet. The only difficulty we had with this piece was the colour of Lucy's dress – the colour is so sharp that it can go dead if you put cold colours on it, and develops a different kind of richness if you put, say, a red-based blue on it. Clear light would have been best but that's not the right treatment for the rest of the work. *Praeludium* is soft and lyrical so I had to keep all the light changes very subtle. I concentrated on emphasizing the mood, rather than imposing a drama.

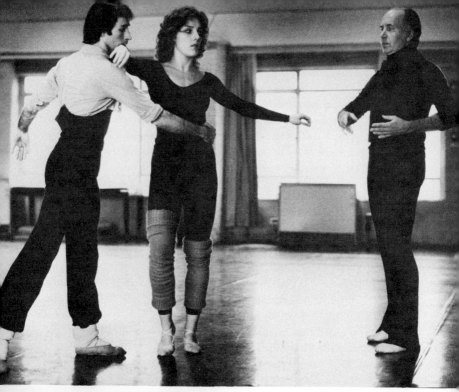

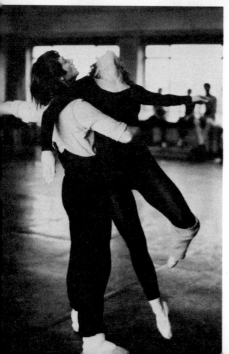

Glen Tetley rehearsing his principals, Lucy Burge and Christopher Bruce, in the sustained *pas de deux* which makes up the core of the ballet. Says Lucy, 'Glen talks about the motivation behind a movement, rather than demonstrating the actual step. He gives an image, and might catch on to some spontaneous gesture a dancer makes, but basically he's very much in command. We don't improvise with Glen. We try to translate the steps he marks out into something fuller.'

Lucy Burge quietly watching her colleagues work. Dancers snatch at any chance to relax during the tension of creating a new ballet. 'This is a difficult role for me,' Lucy explains. 'It's not so hard technically, but it is exhausting to maintain the mood, one of quiet strength, for half an hour.'

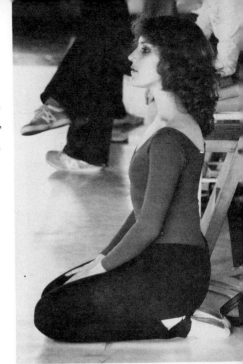

The three other men in the cast struggle to get the high travelling lifts right. Their partners have to concentrate on balancing, and holding their bodies at a particular angle to make themselves as easy to carry and manipulate as possible.

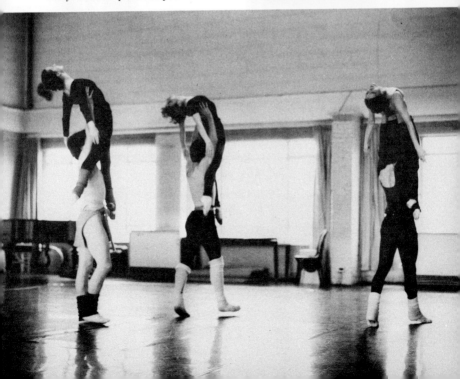

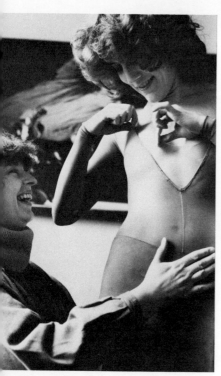

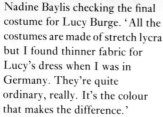

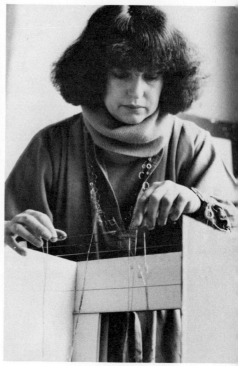

Nadine Baylis checking the final costume for Lucy Burge. 'All the costumes are made of stretch lycra but I found thinner fabric for Lucy's dress when I was in Germany. They're quite ordinary, really. It's the colour that makes the difference.'

The designer with her model, made to a quarter-inch scale. 'The metalworkers curved the tubes and then welded them together in such a way that the whole set could be toured. It's surprisingly light. I use the actual sheen of the metal, instead of painting it over. The whole thing has a very linear quality.'

Dancer Derek Parker being fitted by the company's wardrobe mistress. In the great majority of modern ballets the clothes worn by the performers are extremely form-fitting, some would say revealing, in order to define the movements. The invention of elastic, synthetic fabrics over the past few years means that dancers no longer have to struggle with baggy tights and slipping shoulder straps.

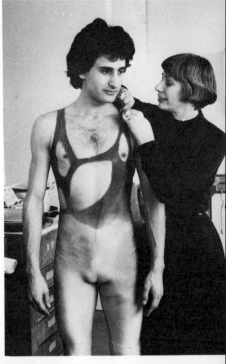

Derek making up before a performance. All members of the cast, and understudies, must be in their dressing rooms by the half-hour call, for even basic make-up such as that being applied by Derek takes fifteen or twenty minutes to put on, and dancers normally do a warm-up exercise session as well.

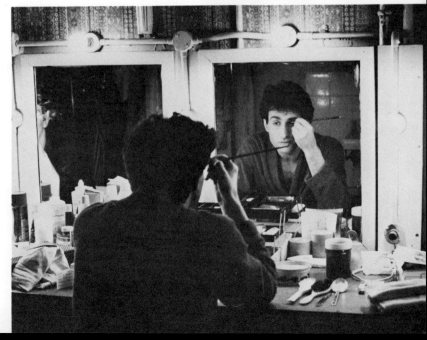

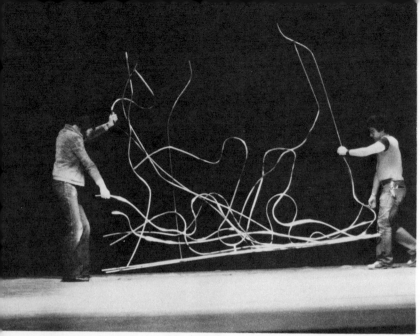

Stage technicians carrying the central piece of Nadine Baylis's set into position.

Dancers hanging about the stage while they wait for the stage–manager and the crew to complete their tasks. There is inevitably a great deal of tedious hanging about in the performer's life, particularly if the company tours a lot. The Ballet Rambert is on the road about five months of every year, both in Britain and abroad.

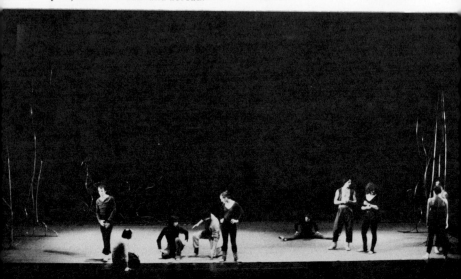

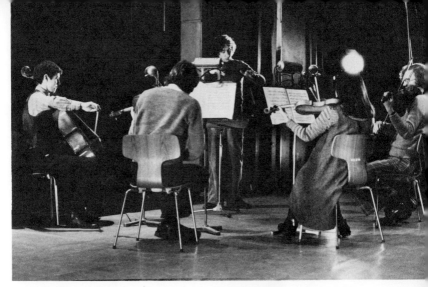

The chamber quartet, members of the company's own Mercury Ensemble, rehearsing the Webern music on stage, with Adam Gatehouse conducting.

Lighting designer John B. Read at the console of the Sadler's Wells Theatre in London, during the final dress rehearsal. Reproduced is an extract from a page of one of his scores, showing how he plots the movements of the dancers and the angles at which the lights should be set. The crosses mark the starting position for the performers in a sequence, while the dotted lines show their progress across the stage. The L represents Lucy Burge and the notes on the sight, 'Warmer tones for couples – poss 61 sp bar' plus 'Get some separation' are Read's personal reminders of his ideas for that section of the work. The arrow indicates the direction of the light.

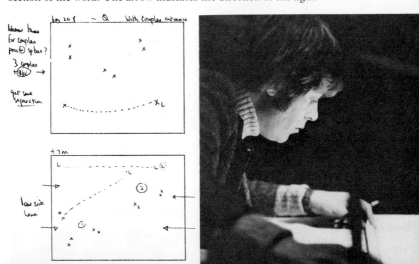

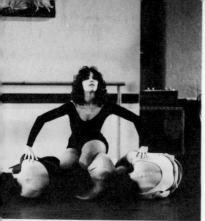

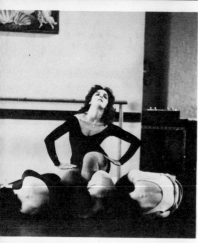

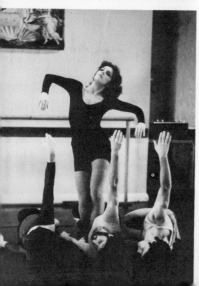

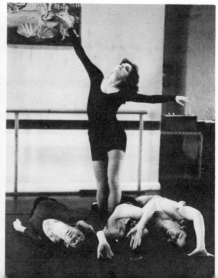

Rehearsal action shots of the opening sequence of *Praeludium*, during which Lucy Burge rises from a trio of recumbent men, her attendants.

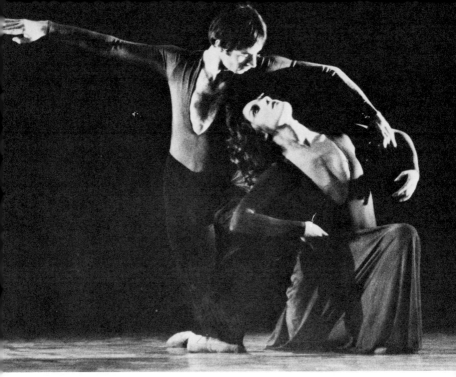

Burge and Christopher Bruce in a typically flowing pose from the ballet. This photo was taken during performance.

One of the final moments of the work, during which Burge displays the strength and serenity of the 'Mother Earth' figure she has played.

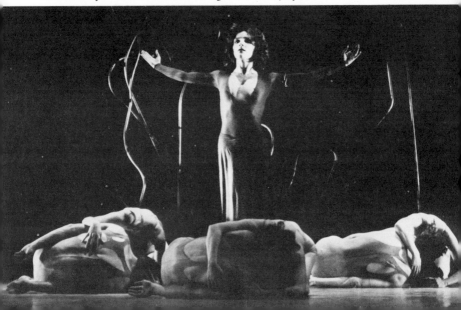

4 · Classical Ballet: The Mainstream

In spite of the impact of modern movers, the general public continues to think of classical ballet as synonymous with theatrical dance. Originating in lavish Renaissance spectacles (the word 'ballet' is derived from the Italian verb *ballare* which means 'to dance') and subsequently taken up by the French court, the professional foundations of ballet were laid down at Louis XIV's Académie Royale de Danse, established in 1661 and shortly afterwards supplanted by a training school – the institution we know as the Paris Opéra – that began to systemize the technique.

Since then the history of ballet has veered between dazzling highs and decadent lows, but because of its essential conservatism, the form has managed to maintain its strict technical framework while adapting to the needs of each new wave of artists. This originally aristocratic entertainment has become sufficiently flexible to depict a woebegone puppet, prisoners in a concentration camp, an older woman ravished by memories of her former loves, revolutionaries and cowboys. Ballet at its best, surviving social upheavals, and incorporating elements of court, folk and modern dance, is, in Lincoln Kirstein's words, 'still an incomparable metaphor of humane possibility'.

From the days when the leading parts were fought over by members of the nobility, ballet has been built on a hierarchical system exemplified by cast lists in modern programmes: principals, soloists, coryphées and, on the bottom rung, the numerous *corps de ballet*. For over a century single performers have been promoted and worshipped until a few have achieved legendary status. Today, superstars are still ballet's most conspicuous asset, the tangible embodiment of flights of fancy. This élitism contrasts strongly with modern dance ensembles, in which even the director/leading dancer may be named alphabetically with the rest of the company.

Beginning with the ethereal Marie Taglioni, who created the title-role of *La Sylphide* in 1832, and through a long line of splendid ballerinas which culminated, this century, in Anna Pavlova, Galina Ulanova and Margot Fonteyn, women have been the focus of balletomanes' affection. There were some charismatic male dancers in the past, too – fans referred to both father and son, Gaetano and Auguste Vestri, as 'the god of dance' – but it was not until Vaslav Nijinsky leapt into international notoriety with the first Paris season of Diaghilev's Ballet in 1909 that men were accepted as major draws at the box office. Two other Russian emigrés have of late been acclaimed with similar fervour, Rudolf Nureyev and Mikhail Baryshnikov, the former born in 1938, the latter ten years later. Between them, they have glorified the position of men in ballet past all recognition. Nureyev is noted for his animal magnetism, terrific range and attack; Baryshnikov, quite simply, is probably the most complete male dancer the world has ever seen.

Superstars of ballet have always been itinerant, aided by the universality of dance language and regular revivals of the same classical works throughout the world. Fonteyn can interpret the role of Giselle with ensembles from Scandinavia to South America, and has probably done so. Pavlova initiated global tours, dragging her supporting troupe to the most remote areas, thereby blazing a trail of inspiration which has had far-reaching effects. Frederick Ashton, for example, the distinguished choreographer who was to become director of the Royal Ballet, was inspired to study dance after seeing a Pavlova performance in Lima, Peru, back in 1917. Today, Nureyev must have clocked up more dance mileage than anyone else, pursuing a frenetic schedule which will see him dashing to the airport minutes after

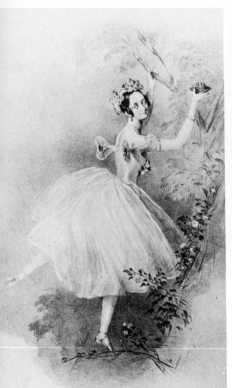

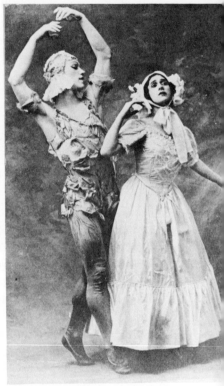

Marie Taglioni in *La Sylphide*, the first 'Romantic' ballet

Nijinsky with his partner Tamara Karsavina in *Le Spectre de la Rose* (1911)

Rudolf Nureyev as a factory cleaner in Toer van Schayk's modern *Faun* for the Dutch National Ballet (Alexandra Radius in the background)

Mikhail Baryshnikov high-kicking his way through a witty solo in Twyla Tharp's *Push Comes to Shove* for the American Ballet Theatre. (He now dances with the New York City Ballet)

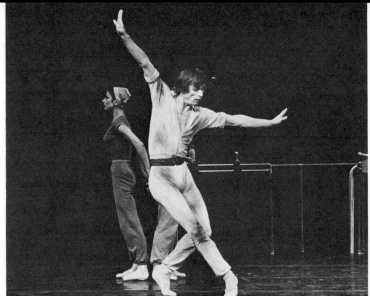

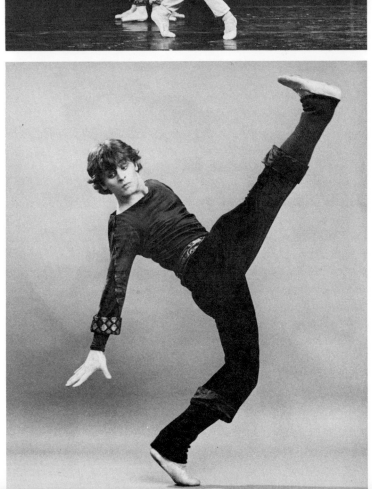

a curtain falls, in order to appear in another theatre on another continent the following night. Stars who stay at home do not become superstars, nor as rich, as those prepared to face the grind of incessant travel.

Except for that quintessentially British ballerina, Fonteyn, Russian dancers have dominated the public imagination. This is no accident for, besides the journalistic capital made from the 'defections' to the west of Nureyev, Baryshnikov, the Panovs and the brilliant Natalia Makarova, these Soviet dancers share a common heritage – an outstandingly effective training system created by Agrippina Vaganova for the dance academy in Leningrad, and extended within that vast country under scrupulous control.

Throughout the world, most establishment companies possess their own schools, and recruit from the graduates, but only in the USSR does the whole weight of government and public approval designate ballet as a uniquely prestigious profession. Thousands of children take part in auditions for the state ballet schools every year, and only the cream are selected. With such resources to draw upon, it is inevitable that dancers who rise to the top in Russia will stay at the top wherever they go. It is relevant that both Nureyev and Baryshnikov have written more warmly of their teacher at the Kirov, Alexander Pushkin, than of any other past colleague.

Fonteyn is therefore doubly exceptional. She has never possessed the virtuoso technique displayed by the Russians and, except for the tragic incident when her husband was seriously wounded by a political opponent, has provided little fodder for the columnists. Like Nureyev and Baryshnikov, she has received the accolade of a *Time* cover story (Baryshnikov, in fact, was featured on *Time* and *Newsweek* the same day, an indisputable proof of fame), but Fonteyn's enduring popularity rests rather on her special qualities of sensitive musicality, a wonderfully limpid line, and quiet dark beauty allied to an authoritative stage presence. She gives a clue to her success in her autobiography:

'I cannot imagine feeling lackadaisical about a performance. I treat each encounter as a matter of life and death. The one important thing I have learnt over the years is the difference between taking one's work seriously and taking oneself seriously. The first is imperative and the second disastrous.'

Natalia Makarova, on the other hand, cannot afford to rest on her laurels. She has serious rivals in Lynn Seymour of the Royal Ballet, who glories in a similar combination of technical and dramatic power, and the young American, Gelsey Kirkland. Another Russian, Nadezhda Pavlova, only made her official début in 1975 and is already causing a stir in dance circles, while Karen Kain from the National Ballet of Canada is caught up in a whirl of international guest appearances. Popular opinion would have it that ballerinas reach a peak in their dewy twenties, but Fonteyn is approaching sixty, and Makarova and Seymour are nearly forty; some dancers have exceptional stamina which enables them to continue performing past normal age limitations. Ballerinas are a notoriously long-lived bunch, although their male partners tend to drop out rather abruptly.

Exposure on television and in feature films is responsible for introducing them to the non-theatre-going masses, an advantage denied their predecessors. The first dance stars of the screen were, of course, the incomparable Fred Astaire and athletic, ebullient Gene Kelly. *The Red Shoes* turned millions of people on to ballet and titian-haired Moira Shearer. By the 1950s important productions by the major companies were being recorded on film, and classics like *Swan Lake*, *The Sleeping Beauty* and *Romeo and Juliet* still do the rounds of art cinemas. A documentary about Nureyev's life-style was disappointing, but it did at least show the taxing routine of a serious dancer. Baryshnikov recently played a character remarkably like himself, in a Hollywood fiction called *The Turning Point*. Unfortunately, with the exception of some imaginative sequences in musicals, movie directors seem to find it impossible to transfer the immediacy and perspective of a live performance on to

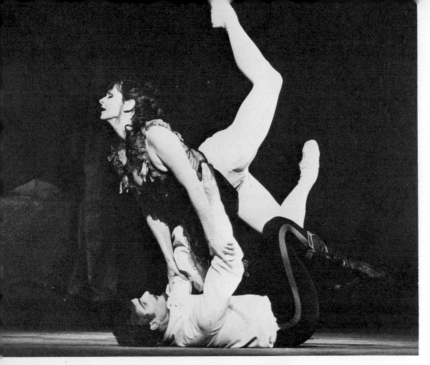

Lynn Seymour with
David Wall in the
Royal Ballet's dramatic
Mayerling by Kenneth
MacMillan (a still from
the award-winning
documentary on the
production made by
London Weekend
Television)

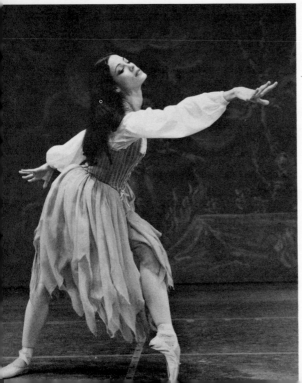

Karen Kain in the
National Ballet of
Canada's *Don Juan*,
choreographed by
John Neumeier

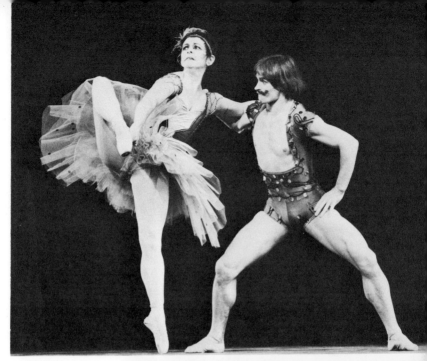

Another side of
Seymour, with
Nureyev in a campy
duet by Kenneth
MacMillan. Seymour
left the Royal Ballet
late in 1978 to direct
the ballet company
of the Bavarian
State Opera in
Munich

Margot Fonteyn in one
of her most famous
roles, Odette in *Swan
Lake*, partnered by
David Wall of the
Royal Ballet

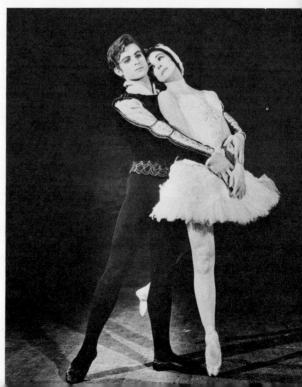

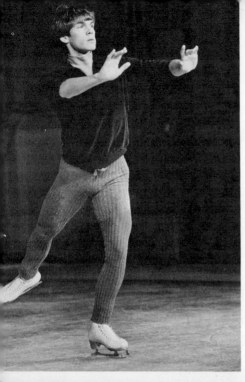

John Curry rehearsing for the first season of his Theatre of Skating

Curry in John Butler's striking *Icarus* with designs by Nadine Baylis

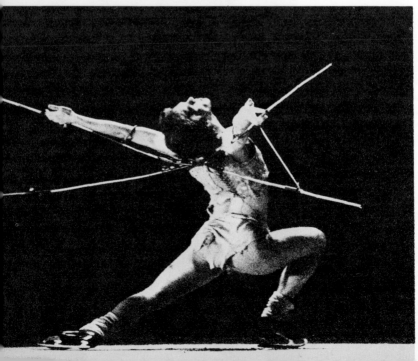

celluloid, so the majority of ballet films are a disservice to the art.

Television programmes have been more successful, particularly those conceived *for* the camera by choreographers Birgit Cullberg, Alwin Nikolais and Twyla Tharp. Both the British and the Canadian Broadcasting Corporations have commissioned documentaries and, in the USA, the Public Broadcasting Service has run an exceptionally fine series entitled 'Dance in America'. Ballet pops up on Dutch and German networks with increasing frequency and experimentalists in video have produced some off beat glimpses of new choreography. Yet the whole field has been circumscribed by union difficulties and lack of adequate financial support and creative exploitation. This is a ridiculous state of affairs given the huge viewing figures for sports like gymnastics and ice skating which share principles of stylized movement with theatrical dance.

At this juncture John Curry should be mentioned, for this British skater, holder of the European, World and Olympic titles in 1976, has done an amazing PR job for dance. Although his parents discouraged him from studying ballet, Curry always thought of skating as ice dancing. In his early teens he began to create solo exhibition pieces, and drew on classical music and dance concepts for his inspiration. It is this choreographic approach, coupled with a near flawless grace, that gains him all his awards. When he came to found the Theatre of Skating, he commissioned ballet choreographers and designers to mount his first programmes, which have since played in traditional theatres with a portable rink laid over the stage.

Curry explains the connection between dance and his chosen sport: 'Anyone who can do an elementary ballet *barre* properly should be able to skate gold figures. The basic positions are so closely related that you could teach one technique in terms of the other. Ballet has helped my line enormously, because I had the typical skater's sway back, while jazz and modern dance emphasize a sense of commitment to movement. Now I make the members of my company take a dance class every day, as I do.'

Russian skaters such as the champion duo Oleg and Ludmilla Protopopov (whom Curry greatly admires) proved the benefits of their ballet training with their graceful high lifts and sustained control in slow passages. Curry has extended the range of skating still further, including in the same evening razzle-dazzle show-stoppers, smoothly balletic pieces and an ambitious duo for himself and a male partner which is very contemporary in style. His Theatre of Skating attracts a heterogeneous public – sports fans, balletomanes, family parties – and is reviewed, most favourably, by dance critics. Now Curry is planning a skating school which will expose students to artistic stimuli rather than concentrating on competitive instincts and the idea that physical skills should be crudely exploited:

The commercial ice shows have a lot to answer for. They sell skating tricks so aggressively that it turns spectators off. I don't know if what I'm doing now with ice dancing is an art form or not, but I do know that I'm trying to develop the essence of skating, if only to satisfy my own inclinations. The difference between the commercial shows and mine is the basic intention and the degree of compromise. I want to explore a mood or an atmosphere, make a statement about the music or movement or shapes. If you're working in the theatre it's important to entertain the audience, yet you shouldn't have to force a reaction by obvious means. Personally, I'm as interested in the process as in the results, and like to bang all the stunts into my first number so that afterwards I can get on with what I really love to do.

The fact that a supreme athlete like Curry is coming to rely on dance choreographers underlines the vital function of these comparatively anonymous artists. In modern dance, the chief choreographer is often the leading performer, as well, but classical choreographers rarely appear in the limelight so their importance is overshadowed by the attention paid to the stars. This is both unfair and illogical, for dancers are only as good as their material (albeit exceptional bodies may convert the dross of flimsy showcases into something approaching theatrical gold) and it is choreographers, sometimes referred to as ballet masters, who have guided the growth of ballet.

Historically, the most famous names are those of August Bournonville, who revitalized the Romantic movement with his version of *La Sylphide*, still preserved in many repertories, and Marius Petipa, who was the architect of the Imperial Russian Ballet and whose productions of *The Sleeping Beauty* and *La Bayadère* are regarded by many as the ultimate tests of a ballerina. His collaborations with Ivanov resulted in *Swan Lake*, the essential 'white' ballet; Ivanov went on to choreograph *The Nutcracker*, although only his final *pas de deux* for the Sugar Plum Fairy and her Cavalier has survived. If *Giselle* and *Coppelia* are added to this list you have a complete line-up of the

La Sylphide in the Royal Danish Ballet's production, with Anna Laerkesen in the title-role and Peter Schaufuss as the young Scot whose life she disrupts

Makarova in the title-role of *Giselle* with Ivan Nagy as her aristocratic lover, in the American Ballet Theatre's version of the classic

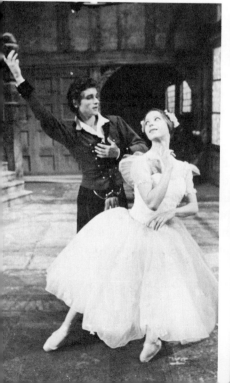
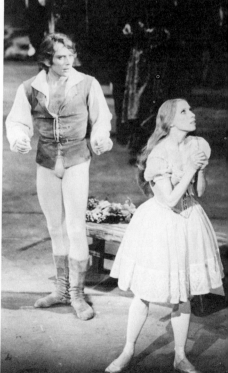

nineteenth-century classics which have provided the basis of the ballet repertory today.

Moving into the present century, the Russian Mikhail Fokine must take pride of place, for he brought the tautly constructed one-act dance drama to its highest level, as well as choreographing the most popular abstract ballet of all, *Les Sylphides*, named in honour of the original Romantic work. He died in America in 1942 but his creations continue to be performed everywhere. The most familiar are *Petrushka* and *Firebird*, both set to original scores by the composer Igor Stravinsky, who has had such a crucial influence on ballet music, and *Le Spectre de la Rose*, which included Nijinsky's immortal exit through a window. This was described, memorably, by the French writer Jean Cocteau: 'He evaporates through the window in a jump so poignant, so contrary to all the laws of flight and balance, following so high and curved a trajectory, that I shall never again smell a rose without this ineffaceable phantom appearing before me.' Of that famous leap Dame Marie Rambert simply says, 'I don't know how far from the ground it was, but I know it was near the stars.'

Fokine was given his opportunities by Serge Diaghilev, the director/impresario who reinstated ballet as a serious entity. His genius at finding and bringing together artists of the first rank from all disciplines make the credits of his Ballets Russes programmes resemble a compilation of the greats of the first three decades of this century: painters like Benois, Bakst, Matisse and Picasso; musicians like Poulenc, Prokofiev and Ravel; choreographers, apart from Fokine, like Nijinsky and his sister Nijinska (her *Les Noces* is rated as one of the masterworks of all time), Massine and Balanchine. To fully appreciate his achievement, it is only necessary to read about the miserable state of ballet at the end of the nineteenth century and go on to study any of the countless documents recording his company's twenty-year history. It makes a gripping tale and is a reminder of the astonishing impact of one forceful mind on a whole genre.

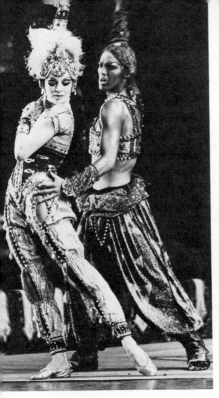

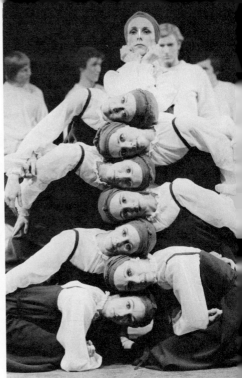

London Festival Ballet's revival of *Scheherezade*, first mounted for Diaghilev's company. Note the sumptuous costumes by Leon Bakst. Dudley von Loggenburg is the Golden Slave, Manola Asensio the Shah's favourite (left)

Nijinska's *Les Noces*, performed by members of Britain's Royal Ballet for a recent BBC television programme. Georgina Parkinson is on top of the pile

One of Pablo Picasso's designs for *Parade*, created for the Ballets Russes in 1917, now performed by London Festival Ballet and the Joffrey Ballet of New York

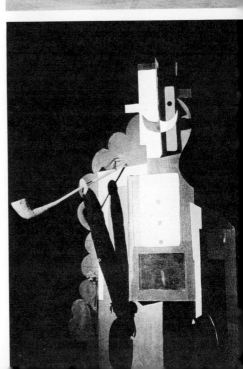

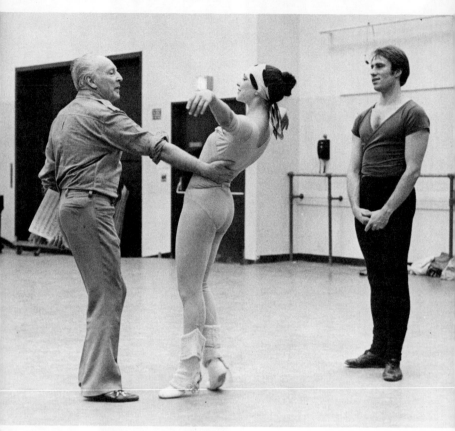

George Balanchine, now a sprightly seventy-five-year-old, rehearsing members of his company, the New York City Ballet

After Diaghilev's death in 1929 the repertory was preserved, in part, by two separate touring companies, but it was left to a handful of Ballets Russes members to maintain the thrust of his legacy. Of these, George Balanchine was to prove much the most important choreographer. Although he was born a Russian, Georgi Balanchivadze, he co-founded the New York City Ballet and there created a body of works that have established a distinctively American style of classicism. His long association

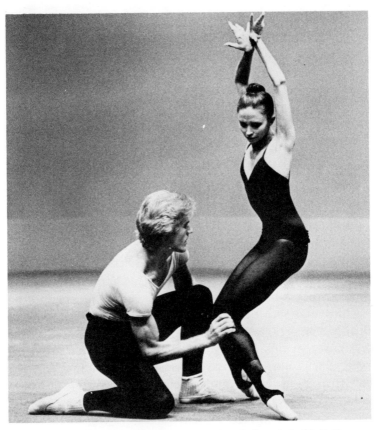

Kay Mazzo and Peter Martins perform Balanchine's *Stravinsky Violin Concerto*, one of the many brilliant collaborations between the choreographer and the late composer. (A still from that fine Public Broadcasting Service TV series in the USA 'Great Performances'.) Along with Anthony Dowell and Fernando Bujones, Martins is considered one of the best classical male dancers in the west

with the composer Stravinsky resulted in seminal creations now presented throughout the world.

It does not require much exposure to ballet to be able to assign Balanchine choreography. His range is wide, his prolificacy formidable (more than one hundred creations), yet the finest works, if one can draw a generalization, are abstract and austere. The favourite Balanchine dancer is long-limbed and svelte, able to deal with the surprising twists and inversions of his vocabulary and, by necessity, extremely musical. The cast is often dressed in simple tights and tunics or T-shirts, the performing area is bare.

Two other Diaghilev products were to found British ballet: Marie Rambert and Ninette de Valois, both dubbed Dame Commanders of the Order of the British Empire (DBE). The former created the Ballet Rambert which, as noted previously, took on a new lease of life when in 1966 it changed from being a medium-sized classical company to an innovative contemporary unit. At that time, Dame Marie was nearly eighty years old, but with typical zest she closely involved herself in new artistic policies, and to this day has never missed an important performance. Rambert has concentrated her remarkable energies on teaching and directing, and fostered the first generation of British choreographers in her tiny theatre in west London. She says now that this is her proudest achievement and given the talents she produced, it is an understandable attitude. Rambert dancemakers included Antony Tudor, the originator of ballets imbued with psychological realism which have confirmed him as one of the most influential dance artists of the century, and Frederick Ashton.

De Valois persuaded Ashton to work with her youthful Vic-Wells Ballet, and by the time the company was granted the Queen's charter and renamed the Royal Ballet, in 1956, Ashton had 'done a Balanchine' and evolved a choreographic idiom that has come to identify the British style. Again, like Balanchine, Ashton has produced a large and varied collection, but his hallmarks are an earthy humour in the comic, story ballets, refined lyricism in the abstract. He has an exceptional gift for choreographing rapturous *pas de deux*, and many a dreary gala event has been enlivened by a gem-like duet of Ashton's.

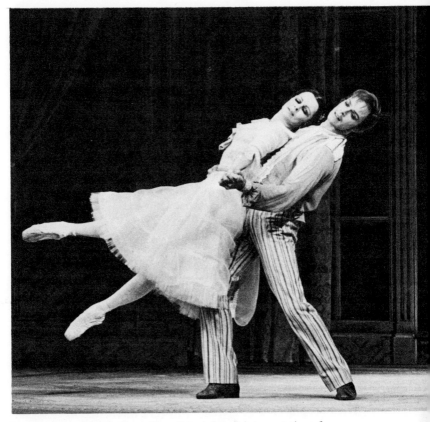

Lynn Seymour and Anthony Dowell in Ashton's interpretation of
Turgenev's play, *A Month in the Country*, for the Royal Ballet of Britain

Ashton succeeded de Valois as director of the Royal Ballet and
he in turn was followed by another choreographer who has made
an international mark, Kenneth MacMillan. Whereas Margot
Fonteyn was Ashton's muse, MacMillan chose 'ballet's greatest
actress', Lynn Seymour, as his main interpreter, and his best
creations have used her extraordinary dramatic abilities. Now it
is Norman Morrice's turn to run Britain's most prestigious com-

pany, and as it was he who guided the Ballet Rambert in a fresh direction, it will be interesting to see whether he will choose to inject new blood into the traditional repertory of the Royal Ballet.

Ashton and Balanchine are the only living ballet choreographers universally acknowledged to be geniuses, but there is another contender for this title, Jerome Robbins. He is without question the foremost American-born classicist, and has developed his gifts without the support of a home company. Indeed, Robbins has made a virtue of his nomadic career, dividing his time between Broadway, where he successfully directed plays and musicals, his production of *West Side Story* being a landmark in theatre history, and pure dance. For a brief period he ran his own company, Ballets: USA, which featured jazz-based dance, but has created the majority of his works on the American Ballet Theatre and, latterly, the New York City Ballet. There is no such thing as a Robbins style, because his spectrum is so wide that at some point or another he has managed to stimulate every imaginable taste.

John Cranko and Maurice Béjart complete the list of choreographers whose ballets are in international demand. Cranko ran the Stuttgart Ballet until his tragically early death in 1973, which robbed the world stage of a vividly theatrical creator. Never enthusiastic about the stereotypes of ballet, he was quoted in a newspaper interview as saying, 'I'm very interested in changing the image of the ballerina as a perpetual virgin and the male dancer as a sort of romantic coat hanger. I want to make it acceptable that a woman can get older.'

Béjart is also something of a renegade, specializing in grandiose multi-media spectacles which sometimes threaten to swamp the dancers. He is regularly slated by critics as being vulgar and pretentious, but his Ballet of the 20th Century, based in Brussels but continually touring, has attracted vast young

---

The Brazilian ballerina Marcia Haydée, now director of the Stuttgart Ballet, with Richard Cragun in Cranko's version of *The Taming of the Shrew*

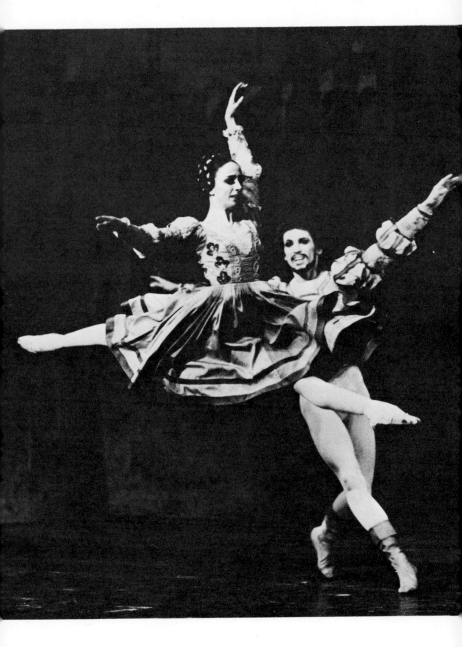

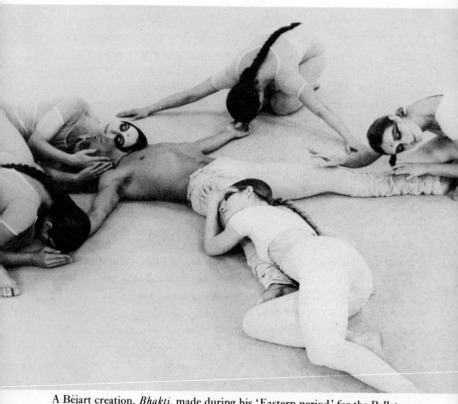

A Béjart creation, *Bhakti*, made during his 'Eastern period' for the Ballet of the 20th Century

audiences to performances in sports stadia and outdoor amphitheatres. His male dancers are some of the most exciting to be found in any company (the women usually play a very secondary role) and his school, Mudra, is one of the most innovative. This centre trains students in all the performing arts and a variety of dance techniques. Supported by UNESCO, it will shortly open a branch in Senegal, the first of several planned to encircle the globe.

The sheer weight of names in this chapter should indicate the volume of activity going on at this moment. Virtually every western country supports one or more national companies, and even Japan, sited far away from the mainstream, has eight classical ensembles. A check-list of the most important would go something like this: the National Ballets of Australia, Canada, Cuba and Holland; the star-studded American Ballet Theatre, the New York City Ballet and the Joffrey Ballet thriving in Manhattan (the USA also boasts a large number of successful regional ensembles); in France, the Paris Opéra Ballet and Roland Petit's Ballets de Marseille; Germany nurtures over fifty opera ballets, of which the most reputable are those in Berlin, Hamburg, Munich and Stuttgart, although the situation is fluid with so much competition around; in Britain the Royal Ballet has two wings, one for national touring, and both the London Festival Ballet and Scottish Ballet have many admirers; in Russia the Bolshoi and the Kirov; each of the Scandinavian countries has at least one respected ensemble, Belgium had three at the last count and Austria is justifiably proud of its Vienna State Opera Ballet. There are interesting classical troupes in South and Central America now, and South Africa makes up for its lack of enthusiasm for modern dance by subsidizing a trio of classical ballet companies.

The majority of these organizations are trying to update their period repertoires with new works that reflect contemporary concerns. But for those diehards who prefer the glitter and unreality of traditional productions, it is a good time to be a balletomane. Never before has there been such generous helpings of superb dancers on offer, and although Ashton and Balanchine are now septuagenarians, there are a few younger choreographers who should ensure that ballet will still be popular for many years to come.

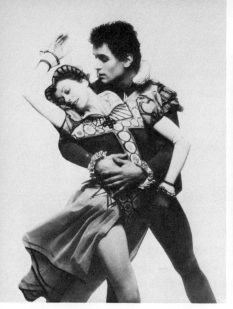

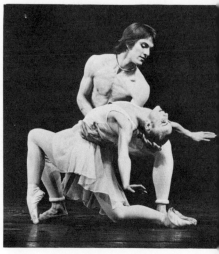

Elaine MacDonald and Graham Bart in their director Peter Darrell's production of *Mary, Queen of Scots* for, appropriately, the Scottish Ballet

Henny Jurriens and Monique Sand in *Adagio Hammerklavier* by Hans van Manen for the Dutch National Ballet

Veronica Tennant, a principal with the National Ballet of Canada, in Roland Petit's work *Kraanerg*, no longer in the Canadian repertory

Dancers of the Asami Classical Ballet of Tokyo, one of several Japanese ballet companies

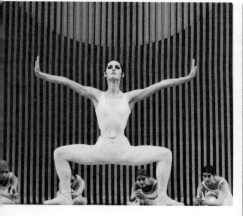

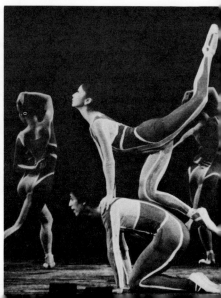

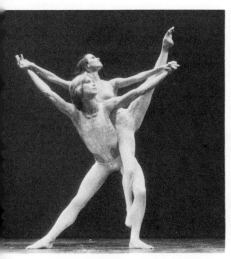

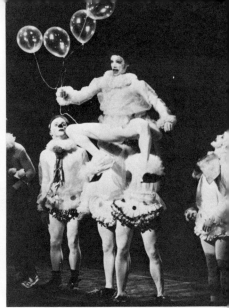

Marielena Mencia and Dale Talley in a
work by American Margo Sappington
for the Ballet Internacional
de Caracas

The Joffrey Ballet in *Clowns*, a highly
theatrical work by the company's chief
choreographer, Gerald Arpino

Jonathan Kelly and Marilyn Jones in
the Australian Ballet's lavish danced
version by Ronald Hynd, of *The
Merry Widow*

Roland Petit with a companionable doll
in his own unconventional production
of *Coppelia* for the Ballets de Marseille
in France

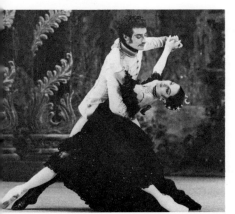

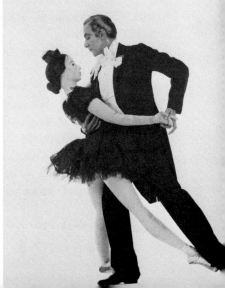

5 · Ethnic Dance

Since time immemorial dance has served many different functions. Curt Sachs wrote: 'On no occasion in the life of primitive peoples could the dance be dispensed with. Birth, circumcision and the consecration of maidens, marriage and death, planting and harvest, the celebration of chieftains, hunting, war and feasts, the changes of the moon and sickness – for all of these the dance was needed.'

With the rise of civilizations dance fulfilled fewer ritualistic purposes. It became a social pastime or entertainment. By the mid twentieth century folk dances began to be valued as living expressions of native culture and professional directors organized theatrical companies to perform choreographed versions of dances people had taken for granted for centuries. This new sophistication meant a loss of authenticity in some cases, but it also brought rich and varied heritages to audiences who would otherwise never witness Zulu warriors preparing for battle, for example, or Balinese girls skimming the stage in intricate patterns.

Dance can speak for an entire nation or race. Today we often refer to these traditional forms as 'ethnic dance' and the two broad areas most in evidence are black dance, whether Afro-American, Caribbean, South American or African, and the highly formal Asian dance theatre. Spanish dance also has great appeal, although people often inaccurately equate it with flamenco which is, in fact, only one of several sources which contribute to Spain's colourful panorama of movement.

The term 'black dance' covers a wide field that is influenced by, or directly expresses, multiple African roots. In the USA black people were largely responsible for the creation of both tap and jazz dancing; there is now a politically conscious type of modern dance associated with black choreographers which American critic Marcia B. Siegel describes as 'the tribal gestures of the ghetto, the assertive upward thrust of the head, and the expressively rotating shoulder, the gliding pelvic step ... these evoke delighted recognition from blacks in the audience, and bemused fascination from whites'.

Alvin Ailey, a Texan born in 1931, is the foremost choreographer working in this milieu. He is proud to be black but does not like to be defined as a black artist. His hugely successful company, the American Dance Theater, is multi-racial and its repertory eclectic; his personal vocabulary embraces jazz, ballet and modern techniques; his choice of music ranges from Negro spirituals through Duke Ellington to the very English Benjamin Britten. Ailey has mounted works for classical companies like the Joffrey Ballet and the American Ballet Theatre; created *Flowers*, about the 'death-trip' of white rock singer Janis Joplin, for ballerina Lynn Seymour; set dances for opera productions. Yet pieces like *Revelations*, the company's signature number which always brings audiences screaming to their feet, the jazz-based *Blues Suite* and the solo *Cry* for his superstar Judith Jamison, which encapsulates the history of black women, could only have come from the Negro experience. Ailey told the author, 'Sometimes I think I should have been a teacher or a politician, so I could say what I want to say about being black. In my dances it's more inference than direct statement, but that's my way of staying out on the streets.'

Other black American choreographers have drawn directly on life in those city streets to produce deeply committed works that can touch or outrage their public. They are fuelled by black consciousness, but produce works that transcend artificial boundaries of colour or creed. They have all been influenced to some extent by the pioneering work of two dancing doctors of anthro-

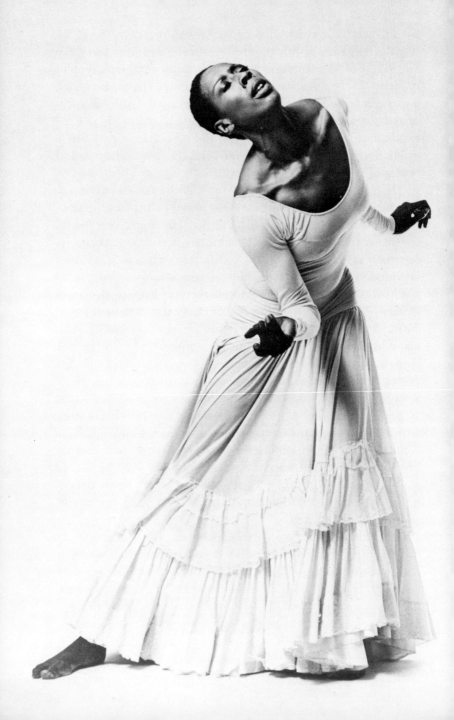

pology, Katherine Dunham and Pearl Primus, who, during the forties, undertook serious research into dances of the Caribbean and Africa, and then incorporated their findings into theatre programmes. Their initiative opened up new opportunities for Negro artists, who had hitherto been confined to music-halls, minstrel shows and cabaret. Primus said, 'When I dance, I am dancing as a human being, but as a human being who has African roots ... I'm learning to deliberately reach beyond the colour of the skin and go into people's souls and hearts and search out that part of them, black or white, which is common to all.'

Arthur Mitchell wanted his people to share another strand of the western heritage, classical dance, so in 1968 he organized ballet classes in Manhattan's Harlem. As the first black principal dancer in a classical company, the New York City Ballet, he had the reputation and the contacts to attract finance and top-flight teachers. Within two years he had assembled a group of young professionals who presented lecture-demonstrations for school-children and, shortly thereafter, full-scale performances. The Dance Theatre of Harlem's repertory is built on classical works, primarily by Mitchell himself or his former director George Balanchine, but includes ethnic pieces inspired by aspects of black culture. Although some critics have questioned the wisdom of introducing contemporary blacks to a white, seventeenth-century court dance form, Mitchell is convinced that the discipline of ballet training is beneficial to everyone. The acclaim which has greeted the company seems to justify his belief, and foreign tours have helped to destroy the prejudice against Negroes in ballet, and the stereotype of hip-swinging, sensu-ously gyrating black dancers. The Harlemites look as poised in *pointe* shoes, as aristocratic in classical variations, as any well-schooled ballet performers. Previously, it had been American contemporary dance that had fostered fine black artists and provided integrated ensembles. Now Mitchell has effectively

The eloquent Judith Jamison in Alvin Ailey's solo *Cry*

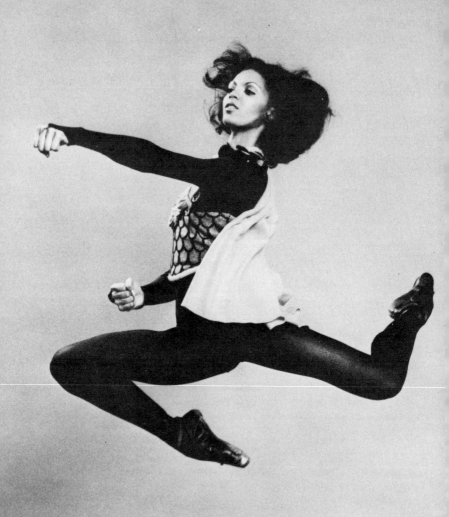

One of the first principals of the Dance Theatre of Harlem, Lydia Abarca, in *Le Combat*

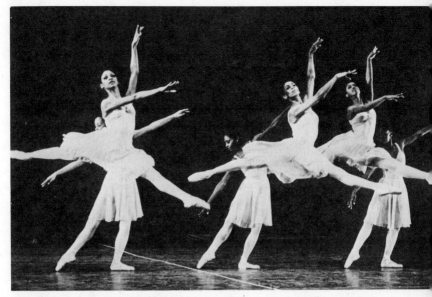

Members of the Harlem Company in *Holberg Suite* by the director, Arthur Mitchell

challenged all those bigots who say 'But you can't have a black swan in *Swan Lake* – it would spoil the effect' or 'Negroes can't dance classical ballet because their bodies are the wrong shape'.

Being located at the crossroads of the slave trade, the Caribbean area absorbed artistic influences from both Africa and Europe, which resulted in a fascinatingly diverse range of dances emerging throughout the islands. Local customs and music are now combined with inherited styles to present diverse portraits of the varied peoples. Trinidad's Folk Performing Company bases programmes on its famous carnival, and includes Indian dances which stem from the country's large Asian population. The National Dance Theatre of Jamaica draws on the cults of *poco* or rastafarianism, while the Danza Nacional de Cuba presents *Yoruba Suite*, which deals with mythological black gods brought by slaves during the period of Spanish colonization.

Reviewing the Carifesta '76, held in Jamaica and involving thirty-five nations from the West Indies and Latin America, an observer noted: 'In such a polyglot culture, one is apt to see an island dance company which combines the restlessly energetic torso found in African dances with the mannered and carefully studied patterns of a European ballroom dance such as the mazurka.' Modern dance techniques, particularly those of Martha Graham, are now taught throughout the Caribbean, and important historical research is being carried on in Trinidad, Haiti and Jamaica. West Indians have preserved traditional social dances that would have otherwise been lost and evolved indigenous forms with a vitality and flavour all their own. A British outpost is currently being established by a group of young black dancers who wish to explore their Afro-Caribbean heritage. Operating under the auspices of the Minorities Arts

Dancers in Britain's black group, the MAAS Movers, rehearsing an ethnic work based on Trinidadian rituals by co-director Evrol Puckerin (the bald gent in the background). The other director, Greta Mendez, is rigorously in the foreground

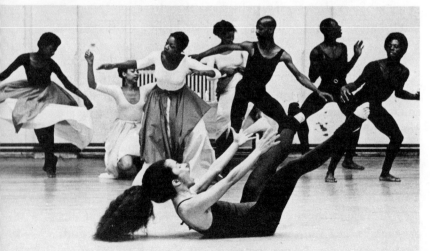

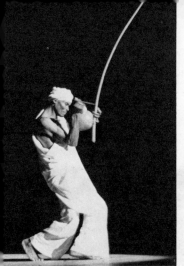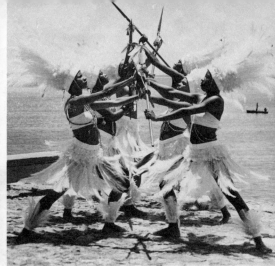

(Left) A Brazilian playing the *berimbau*, which traditionally accompanies the extraordinary dance-martial art form called *capoiera*

(Right) Bahian dancers in a reconstruction of an Amerindian dance from Brazil

Advisory Service – MAAS – this professional black dance ensemble is known as the MAAS Movers.

Further south, Argentina and Brazil boast several accomplished ballet companies, but within the general frame of folk or ethnic dance, the best known groups have come from the predominantly black Brazilian state of Bahia and its capital Salvador. A unique feature of their programmes is the acrobatic dance-fight called *capoeira*, which was developed by runaway slaves in the sixteenth and seventeenth centuries and is still accompanied by an Angolan gourd 'harp', the *berimbau*. This strange martial art form is mostly conducted upside down, with the competitors using wide, slashing kicks (in more vicious times razor blades were placed between the toes) to defeat opponents, while doing head-stands, hand-stands and cart-wheels. *Maculele* dance-combats, with huge bush-knives, resemble Trinidadian *kalinda* or stick-fighting dances, while the familiar samba echoes the joyous rhythms of Caribbean forms like the rumba and conga. The African connection is obvious.

In recent years the African dance groups which have toured most widely have come from the western side of the continent:

A lament over a dead girl in a dance programme from Ghana. The witch doctor is attempting to restore her to life

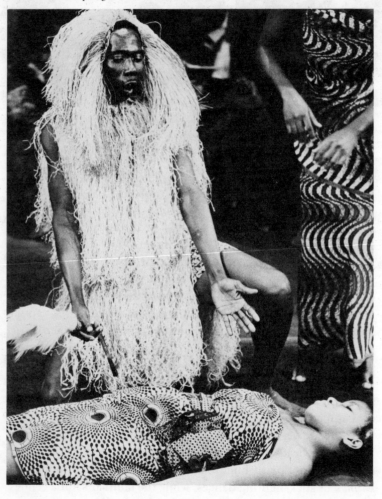

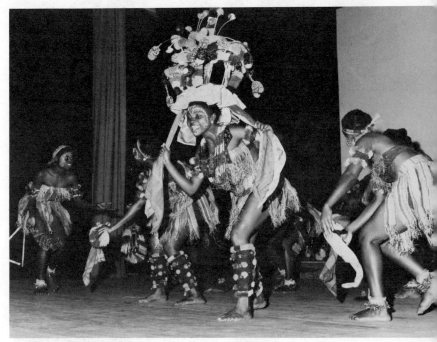

Young Nigerians performing a lively celebration dance

Ghana, Guinea, Nigeria and Senegal. In 1935 a young English-
man, Geoffrey Gorer, travelled through those parts and noted
that 'It is very difficult for Europeans to understand the place
dancing takes in Negro lives. They dance for joy and they
dance for grief; they dance for love and they dance for hate;
they dance to bring prosperity and they dance to avert calamity;
they dance for religion and to pass the time.'

With the upheavals in African life during the past decades
dance is no longer the central means of expression, but the
glories of the native styles continue to enrich international
cultural life. The movement idioms are varied, the themes
rooted in so many different tribal traditions that it is impossible
to generalize about African dance.

133

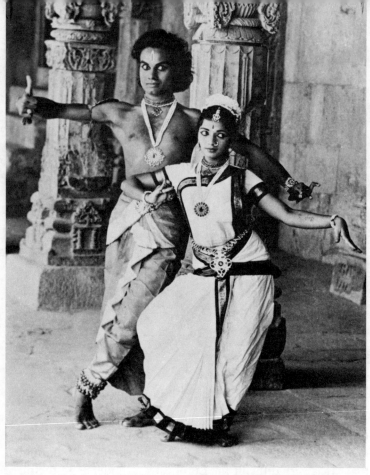

Radha and Raja Reddy, Kuchipudi dancers from India, outside an ancient temple

In its earthiness and percussive complexity, above all in its free use of the entire body, African dance has had a profound influence on contemporary movement in the west. The same could be said of Indian classical dance. Martha Graham drew ideas from Hindu art, ballerina Anna Pavlova collaborated with Uday Shankar, elder brother of the famous sitar player Ravi, to introduce Indian dance into her performances, and Maurice Béjart has created modern ballets, like his *Bhakti*, which utilize

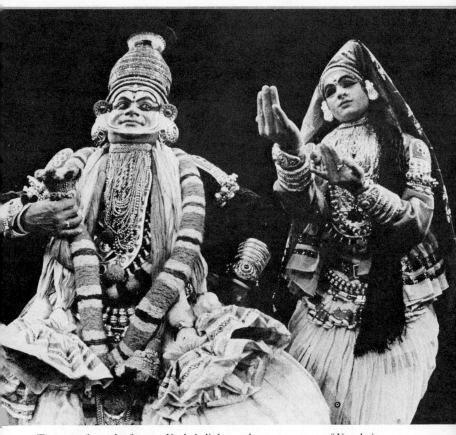

Two men from the famous Kathakali dance-drama company of Kerala in south India

Indian music and philosophy. As western interest in yoga and meditation techniques has grown, and Indian classical music is studied even by pop groups, there is a new, serious audience for the refined and spiritual dances of the Far East.

The classical styles of the India-Pakistan-Bangladesh sub-continent have been absorbed by other countries of eastern Asia. Some are solo forms, some group, but most share a common grounding in the Hindu religion and the canons of a book about dance, drama and music called the *Bharata Natya Shastra*, dated variously from the second century BC to the third century AD. Over hundreds of years a range of virtuoso techniques have been developed, differentiated by the regions in which they originated.

Eastern training methods seem almost brutal to the outsider. Youngsters are expected to dedicate themselves to dance from about the age of twelve, and tuition goes on almost round the clock for more than a decade. A typical schedule of a student of Kathakali (a dance form from southern India) would start at 3 a.m. and would go something like this, at least during the cool, rainy season: gymnastics and physical exercises, followed by a strenuous oil massage, for which the instructor uses his feet – not a comfortable procedure; a nippy plunge into the local river; rehearsal of the repertory until noon; academic studies during the afternoon and, throughout the evening, gesture and acting classes, prayer and singing; to bed by 10 p.m., if possible. The survivors of this intensive apprenticeship possess the most finely attuned physical and nervous systems imaginable. Indian dancers can control and manipulate parts of the body, like the eyes, neck and knuckles, which are virtually ignored in western dance forms. As sections of the choreography are improvised, performers must react immediately to any variations in the musical accompaniment. But with all this personal striving, Indian dance is not ultimately concerned with self-expression. The Hindu god Shiva is called Nataraja, 'Lord of the Cosmic Dance', and dancers are his servants, who interpret his sacred edicts through their art. Even today every dance theatre performance must begin with an invocation to the deity and, usually, the performer's guru.

A newcomer to Indian dance will first be struck by the opulent costumes, jewellery, headgear and make-up. In the case of Kathakali, the traditional garments are so strange and overpowering that it is difficult to concentrate on the action at first. The faces of the male performers (very few women learn this style) are painted symbolically in green, scarlet, yellow, black or white, and further transformed by intricate designs, their eye-balls are tinted red, the jaw is exaggerated by layers of stiffened paper or a beard, a false nose may be added, and the weird result is surmounted by a towering headdress. The body is enlarged, too, by heavy pleated skirts, elaborate chest pieces, jewelled girdles and talon-like nails attached to the left hand. The ulti-mate effect is superhuman, as befits interpreters of gods, heroes and demons (types rather than specific characters) and the prolonged make-up session is used by the actor as a time of deep concentration, during which he is 'taken over' by his role.

Although Kathakali is the most spectacularly dressed of the various classical styles, all the eastern dance forms involve beautiful apparel and complex, stylized gestures of the hands and eyes. This mime language can express names, verbs, tense, full sentences, moods and states of being – a remarkable range of silent communication. The pulse of Indian dance is often slow and stately, with the performer taking up statuesque poses reminiscent of the wonderful sculptures still to be seen in the ancient temples. Though they should not feel that they have to understand the meaning of every gesture, westerners generally require some advance knowledge, or at least the ability to con-centrate on the exquisite movement patterns, in order to enjoy their first exposure to these forms. Indian classical dance theatre can yield great treasures to those with the patience and imagina-tion to follow a timeless ritual.

Unlike Hinduism, the Muslim religion does not recognize dance as a form of worship but there is one Islamic sect, the Sufi brotherhood, which follows a strange dance rite: under the more familiar name of Whirling Dervishes these monks sometimes present their danced ceremony in theatres, and have recently visited western countries. Now based in Turkey, the order was founded in the thirteenth century by a mystic named Mevlana Jalalu'ddin Rumi, who wrote, 'Whosoever knoweth the power of the dance, dwelleth in God.' The dervishes, dressed in long

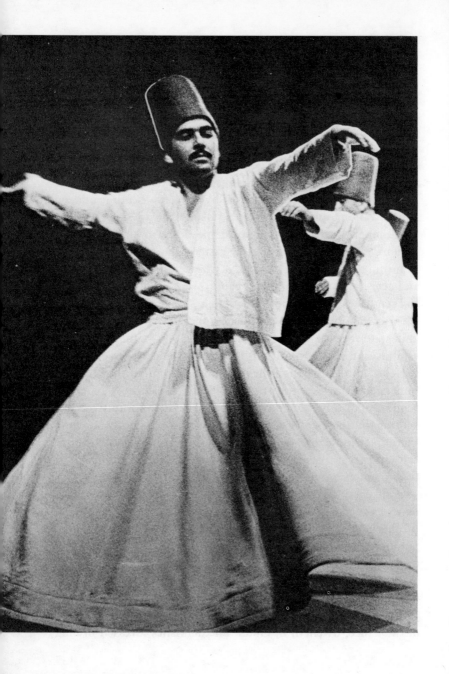

white robes and high conical hats, slowly revolve, sometimes on the spot, sometimes moving in a great circle, the right hand held up to receive Divine Grace, the left palm facing downwards to transmit it to the earth. They can spin like this for an extended period, altering their state of consciousness and transcending the feeling of dizziness to reach a heightened sensation of union with the Eternal. Apparently there were whirling dances in all the countries bordering the Mediterranean in ancient times. The Mahalli dancers of Iran also include the stylization of a dervish ritual in their performances.

Japanese culture is the source of magnificent dance and dance-drama forms, which are still performed locally and toured internationally. The centuries old court dances called Bugaku, the austere classical dance theatre of Noh, and the popular Kabuki tradition all have a large public, while folk dances (the most famous is the masked lion dance) are practised in clubs and at public festivals. The virtuoso percussionist Stomu Yamash'ta with his Red Buddha Theatre and the 'demon' drummers and traditional dancers of the Ondeko-Za group have both proved enormously popular with young western audiences.

The classical dance of China is part of a composite theatre art, the opera, and has exerted considerable influence on neighbouring countries like Korea. Communist Chinese performers visit the west with programmes that combine highly developed and spectacular acrobatics with masked dances and, occasionally, a restricted range of western ballet techniques harnessed to crude political sloganeering. The Koreans have ancient masked dances, too, and a troupe of youngsters called the Little Angels of Korea and the Korean National Dance Company have delighted overseas audiences with the precise, graceful manoeuvres of their group numbers. Many of their dances are based on Buddhist legends and rituals and, unusually in the east,

A whirling dervish

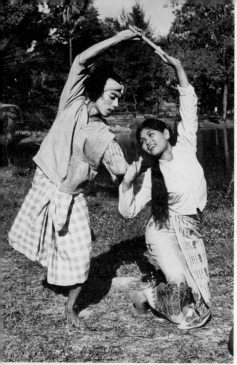

ORIENTAL DANCERS

(Left) A dancing couple from Burma

(Right) A soloist from Bali interpreting the role of Ramayana, in a traditional Hindu story

(Below) Masked Korean dancers with a friendly 'lion'

(Below right) A modern star of Kabuki, Ennosuke Ichikowa, as a man-eating demon

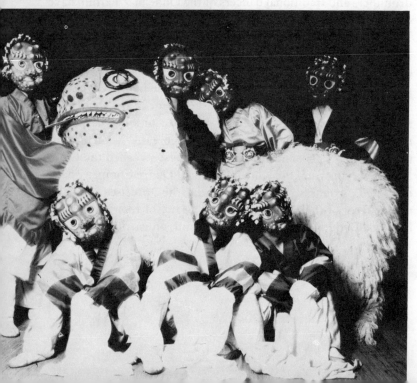

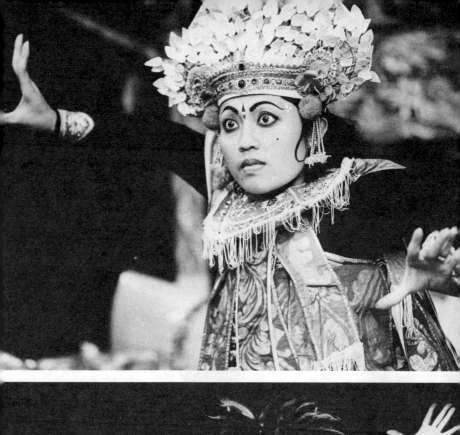
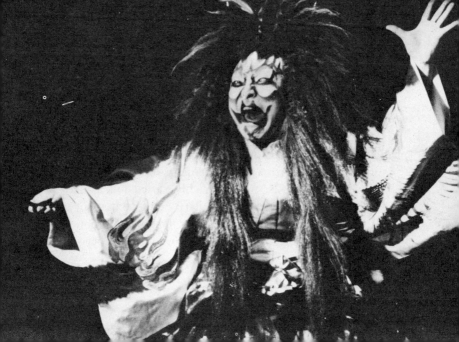

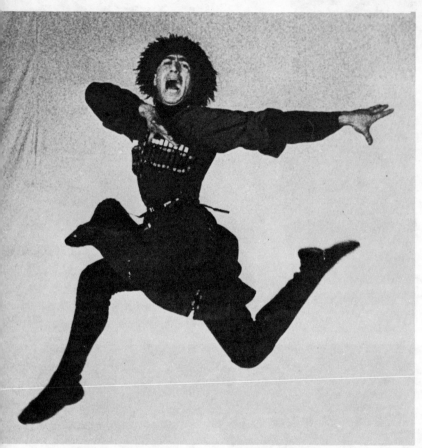

Typically meteoric leap by a Moiseyev dancer

women often predominate. (In dance-drama forms like Kabuki and Kathakali the female roles are played by highly accomplished masculine impersonators who are trained for many years to imitate the mannerisms and movements of the opposite sex.)

Travelling westwards, we find richly varied folk dances in the USSR, where they vie in popularity and excitement with the Russian classical ballet. The most famous folk company was founded by Igor Moiseyev in 1936, and its repertory of more than three hundred numbers awakened foreign audiences to the wonders of social dances developed and polished to the highest level of professional entertainment. The Moiseyev men dance on the toes of their supple, leather boots, spin, leap and strike sparks off each other's swords, while the women have developed a smooth, gliding walk that makes them move as if on roller skates. No simple peasants, these, the dancers undergo arduous training in state schools and their costumes are dramatic and sumptuous. Such has been the success of the Moiseyev ensemble that folk groups from all over eastern Europe now undertake tours around the globe.

Dance in Spain is much more fragmented as, until the formation of the National Dance Company of Spain in 1973 professional presentations were left to the efforts of individual stars. (Only Barcelona's Teatro Liceo has a resident dance company.) Troupes led by famous dancers like 'La Argentina', Pilar López, José Greco, Antonio with his cousin Rosario, Carmen Amaya and Antonio Gades, have taken classical and regional Spanish dance, and the inevitable flamenco, to an adoring public the world over. The chatter of castanets, the fiery stamping of high heels, the swirl of ruffled skirts and propulsive rhythms of a guitar spell Spanish culture to most people. Spanish themes and choreography are used in many classical ballets such as *Don Quixote*, but, because of the lack of government subsidy, much of the splendour of the Iberian tradition – the famous bolero dancing, for example – has been endangered. Tourists think they are seeing 'the real thing' when they visit night clubs and taverns, but too often the dancing is glossy and superficial, designed to appeal to the lowest common denominator rather than express the *duende* or spirit of Spanish art. Permanent employment for dancers is rare, and they must depend on erratic seasons at home and short-term tours abroad for a livelihood.

Iberian dance is multi-faceted, but undoubtedly the most celebrated form is the gypsy flamenco from Andalucia. It is generally accepted that gypsies began to settle in Spain during

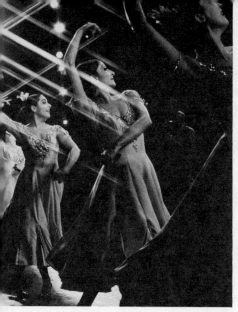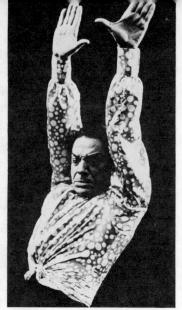

Members of the Ballet Nacional Festivale de España, with castanets

Antonio, one of the great names in Spanish dance, in an authentically impassioned pose

the fifteenth century, but their country of origin remains obscure. Illiterate and nomadic, the gypsies, or *gitanos* as they are known in Spain, assimilated aspects of Andalucian folklore (which had in the past been influenced by Jews, Moors and Arabs) with their own heritage, to produce a superb collection of dances such as the *bulerias*, *farruca* and *zapateado*. The eastern influence is clear in the proud, upright stance, flexible wrists and intricate footwork of flamenco dance, and the sensuality should be dignified and controlled rather than vulgar.

In Greece, too, folk dance is a living tradition and companies like that of Dora Stratou and small ensembles organized by the Lyceum Club of Athens perform abroad, as well as giving

Greeks in the tradional man's costume called *fustanella*

A carnival dance from Macedonia in northern Greece, complete with masks. (It is fascinating how many different cultures incorporate masked dances)

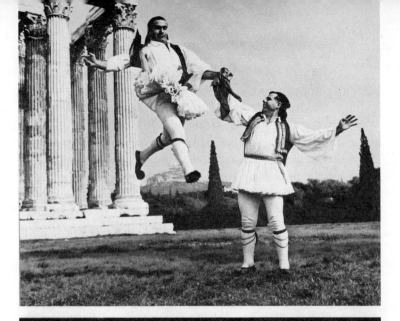

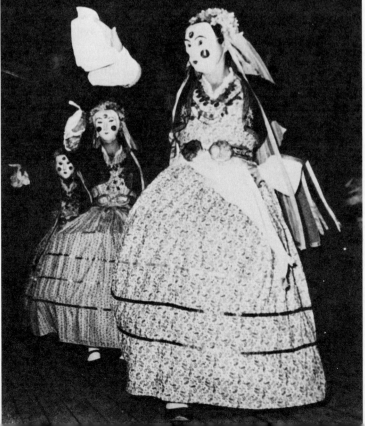

regular shows during the winter and the tourist season. But, as visitors to that beautiful country know, authentic folk dance can be enjoyed in many tavernas, on the mainland and the islands, accompanied by small musical groups – in the cities the bouzouki is usually the dominant instrument, while in the villages it is more often a wind instrument like a clarinet or a violin playing the lead. The film *Zorba the Greek* popularized a dance called the *syrtaki* (really the *khasapiko*) but that is only one of an uncharted number of participatory forms, structured by a variety of complex rhythms. In a technical dance manual Ted Petrides explains the basic differences in stylistic expression:

Although a few are flirtatious or humorous, most Greek dances are serious. The dancers move much as they walk. Mountaineers move proudly and use simple, firm steps combined with leaps; inhabitants of the plains and valleys have more digging, stamping and running steps with a tendency to lean forward or backwards in the direction of the movement; islanders are bouncy and lilting in their movements; city folk have a stealthy character to their steps. In addition, men are expansive in the movements and women restricted.

More and more people are looking to ethnic dance forms to recover the source of their own culture or recreate traditions which affirm the individuality, as well as the common humanity, of races and nations. The magnificent multiplicity of movement styles which can be seen on the stages of larger cities, and are taught in schools and studios everywhere, are beginning to fulfil that primal need.

6 · Experimental Dance

'Anything goes' is a refrain echoed by many contemporary artists, and dance experimentalists are no exception. What is now presented and tolerated as theatrical dance has little connection with the popular image, whether of ballerinas in fluffy tutus or lithe, muscular modernists in leotards. 'New' dancers may be garbed in street clothes, boiler suits or layered variations of rehearsal gear. They may hang from a ceiling and walk on the wall, explore space from a perch on a trapeze, thunder over a basketball court or dodge through rooms in an art gallery. Their movements may be indistinguishable from everyday activities, they may talk throughout an event or encourage the audience to make suggestions on how a dance should proceed. Film, video screens, props of amazing variety, sculptures and live musicians are all incorporated into choreography, and members of the public may end up participating in a group number. In short, our perceptions about what dance should be have changed so radically over the past fifteen years that the experts are still groping for definitions.

So many exponents of the new dance are concerned to bring their work to the community that, ironically, these saboteurs of tradition may be more accessible than touring productions of *Swan Lake* or *The Nutcracker*. Because they reject the conventional proscenium stage they can be found in unexpected places. Admission charges are minimal or non-existent. A performance may be introduced by a lecture-demonstration or an open class so that spectators have the chance to try dance steps themselves, or discuss the concept behind a work with the

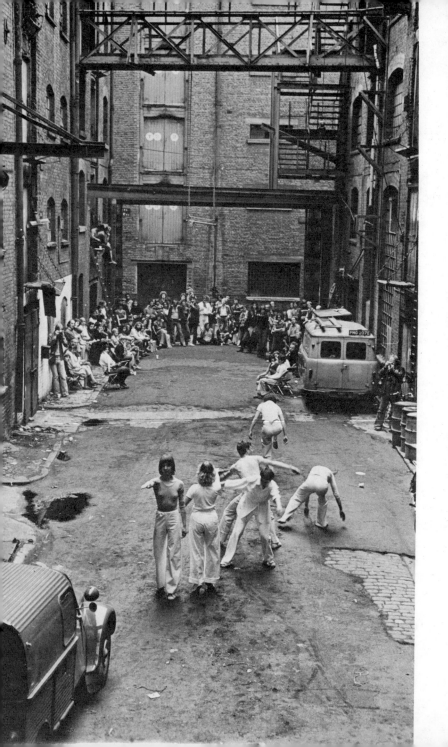

UNEXPECTED ENVIRONMENTS

(Left) A London street: members
of Rosemary Butcher's Dance
Company
(Right) A London square at lunch-
time: Sue MacLennan, Dennis
Greenwood and Miranda Tufnell
(Middle) Water: members of
Trisha Brown's Company from
New York floating happily
(Bottom) Field: Mary Fulkerson
of Dartington College in England

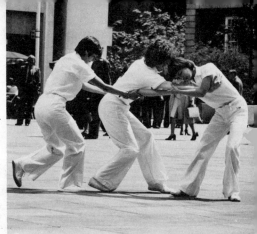

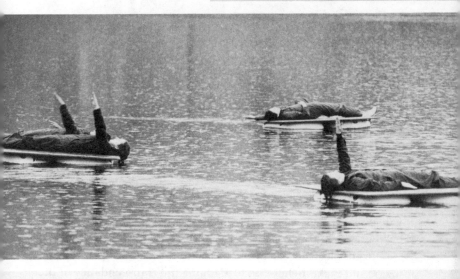

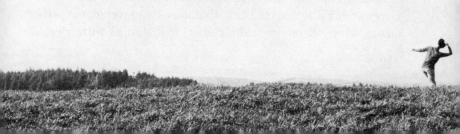

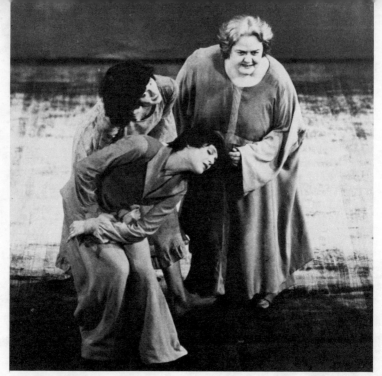

'Anybody of any shape': Margaret Beals (foreground), Brooke Myers and Lee Nagrin (right) in a work inspired by Sylvia Plath's poetry, *Stings*

choreographer. On other occasions a general question period will be held after the programme, for the same purpose. The current generation of radicals is determined to de-mystify dance.

'No to spectacle no to virtuosity no to transformations and magic and make-believe no to glamour and transcendancy of the star image ... no to style no to camp no to moving or being moved', proclaimed Yvonne Rainer, a front-runner of the iconoclastic group which rejected the achievements of its modern dance predecessors as thoroughly as those founders had previously rejected the tenets of classical ballet. This group established the Judson Dance Theater in a church in New York's Greenwich Village in 1962 as a laboratory for movement experiments. Most of the original members had studied with Merce

Cunningham. Painters, sculptors, film-makers and musicians became involved in their chaotic activities. There was no money to subsidize performances (audiences were asked only to make contributions) so everyone had to pitch in and help with stage management, publicity, all the myriad jobs surrounding the presentation of new works. It was a period of intense questioning and of interchanges among all the art forms. Individuals without any dance training found themselves sharing the floor with professionals who had danced with Cunningham's prestigious company. Traditions were bypassed, rules were broken and a whole area of dance re-thought and redefined.

The most revolutionary aspect of the Judson operation was the use of natural or 'found' movement which ignored all technical dance skills. Amplified games and improvisation were emphasized – play rather than polish. Rainer choreographed the smooth, uninflected *Trio A* for example, and taught it to large numbers of people, dancers and non-dancers, who sometimes mingled in a performance. As simple actions like standing or sitting look different when done by different bodies, the Judson artists explored the theatrical possibilities offered by this pedestrian material. Dancers no longer had to be superhuman: they could be anybody, of any shape and age. An artist lurked within everyone.

Currently, this open-ended approach is evidenced in the popular contact improvisation, a form of movement expression

British contact improvisers trained by Steve Paxton

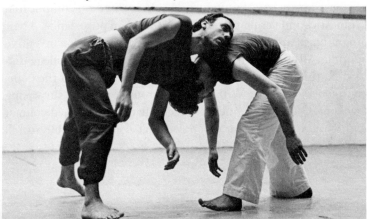

developed by Steve Paxton, one of the Judson founding members. It looks a bit like non-violent martial art or cheerful wrestling, and can have a therapeutic effect on practitioners. Contact improvisers work in pairs, usually, having matched themselves as closely as possible in height and weight. They lope around the floor then come together to roll over each other's backs and hips, intertwine limbs, bounce off one another only to collide again with varying degrees of force. Partners must trust each other, for the spontaneous movement patterns and exchanges of weight develop from wordless communication and confidence that one will support or rescue the other. Accidents can happen, but as the pace tends to be slow and the bodies relaxed, physical damage is rare.

A practitioner describes her reaction to this form:

What I find exciting about contact is the amount of physicality it allows you to achieve in a comparatively short period of time. A great sense of your body, a kind of unconscious grace, like an athlete. For me, a great deal of confidence as well. There also isn't that pressure on you to 'get it right' as there is in other techniques. The body is free to develop at its own pace and, as a result, seems to develop much faster.

The growing connection between certain sports and dance is more dramatically exemplified by the work of a collective called Pilobolus. This group was created by a quartet of male undergraduates at Dartmouth College but by 1973 had assimilated two women who, in contrast to the originators, had extensive dance training. Together these young people have created a repertory of marvellously entertaining works, often based on complicated gymnastics and acrobatic routines rather than pure dance. Their programmes are highly theatrical, in part because of inventive lighting. All the men had been keen athletes, but in college discovered they preferred movement for its own sake to the competitiveness of sport. With this background, it is not surprising that some Pilobolus sequences resemble choreographed contact improvisation, bodies so entangled that it is impossible to tell

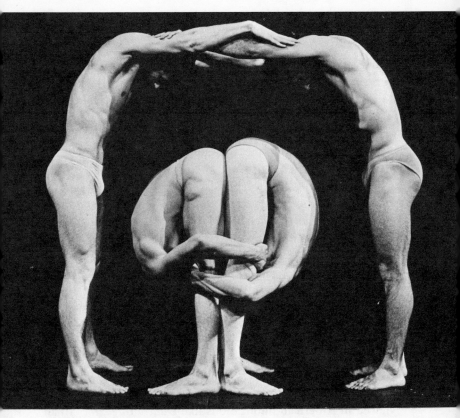

Pilobolus Dance Theatre in gymnastic action

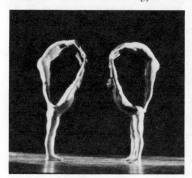
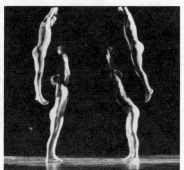

who owns which head or foot, and there is the same emphasis on mutual trust and responsibility.

With the shift from strictly organized companies to the free flow of casual, individualistic events, there have come to be three main performing units amongst experimental dancers: soloists, who often invite the public to their own lofts or studios; co-operatives, like Pilobolus, in which responsibility is shared; and small companies informally grouped around a central teacher or choreographer. Programmes or 'umbrella' seasons are often divided among varied artists and their followers, and the result can be a confusing and/or stimulating jumble of impressions. When the traditional expectations of an audience are over-thrown, the reaction may be boredom or bafflement. But there is no questioning the impact of the revolutionaries on how we look at dance today, and their fascinating experiments with film and sound, objects and locale, the use of real' time (as opposed to artificial theatrical time), mixed-media and speech have subtly infiltrated even the most traditional companies – in the west, at least.

A roll-call of these contemporary pioneers would go on for pages. Their activities have been closely documented by American critics Deborah Jowitt, Don McDonagh and Marcia B. Siegel in engrossing books, and performances are regularly reviewed in American publications like *Dance Magazine*. In an attempt to trace the dissemination of these rebellious theories it might help to look at new dance in Britain, for Britain can be seen as something of a clearing house for innovation, susceptible to both American and continental European influences, yet maintaining a degree of independence.

The contribution made to the rise of modern dance in the UK by both the converted Ballet Rambert and the London Contemporary Dance Theatre has already been discussed in Chapter Three. Some of the earliest experimental events were staged at the home of the latter company, The Place, in the early seventies and included collaborations between sculptors and dancers, multi-media pieces, and visits from controversial artists of all disciplines from many different countries. In those days the building also housed contemporary music ensembles and cinema clubs, and the 'total' theatre group called Moving Being, so the resident students and performers were bombarded with stimuli from every direction. The result was an upsurge in choreographic activity and, before long, a rejection by some dancers of the Graham-orientated approach of the company and its associated school.

Along the way, the obsession with breaking down barriers between art forms has receded, and now most exponents of 'new' dance are concerned with examining the basics of movement, exploring space, time, stillness and weight.

In performance, choreography by these radicals looks stark, and recognizable dance steps may be minimal. Scant use is made of elaborate visual or musical aids, although the setting or environment (occasionally outdoors) is reflected in the movement. The swinging sixties have given way to the subdued seventies, and today's young dancemakers, in Britain at least, seem more concerned with the socio-political relevance of their dance activities or pure art than with theatrical or surprising presentation. They do not want to exhibit flashy skills or communicate private emotional experience, at least not directly.

Excerpts from discussions among alternative movers give an idea of their current preoccupations. The following quotations are taken from the quarterly magazine *New Dance*, published in London, or seminars organized by the X6 collective and ADMA, the Association of Dance and Mime Artists, which was set up as a lobby for the interests of anti-establishment groups.

I am only now, after fifteen years' involvement with dance, discovering how and from where I initiate, sustain and control my movements. During my early years of dance training I had a clear image of what the end product should look like, even what it should feel like, and I worked my body to achieve that image in a state of fearful external

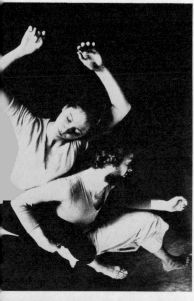

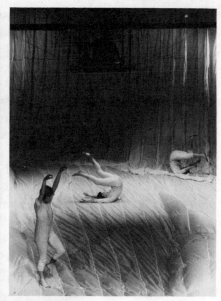

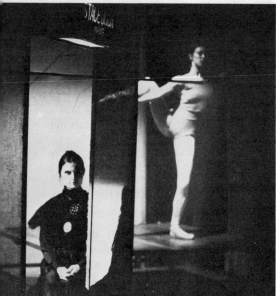

(Top left) Nanette
Hassell and Richard
Alston performing with
Strider, the first
experimental dance group
to be established in
Britain, directed by Alston
in the early seventies

(Above) Members of the
X6 collective, plus
parachute silks, in a
production called
Oceanflight

(Left) The pioneering
mixed-media group
Moving Being in an early
production *Dreamplay*

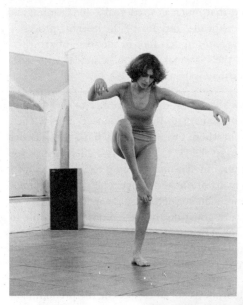

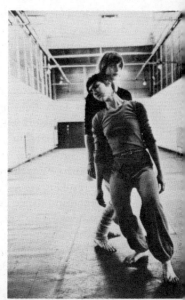

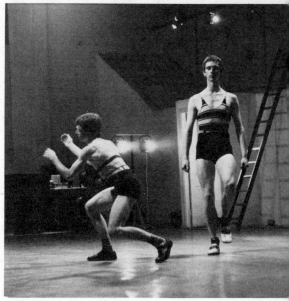

(Above) British soloist
Janet Smith dancing in an
art gallery. The spectators
were impressed

(Above right) Martha
Grogan and Miranda
Tufnell in an
'environmental' event.
The spectators were
confused

Julyen Hamilton (left) and
Timothy Lamford at a
Festival of New Dance and
and Mime in London,
exploring 'the role of men
in dance'

discipline. I never reached that much desired goal – like a mirage it always stayed a little further ahead – and during the learning process I developed permanent damage to my left foot in the form of arthritis. (From a past member of the National Ballet of Canada, who subsequently studied with Martha Graham.)

In New York right now there is a limited number of people who actually want to work with movement itself, so few dancers are stretched physically. It got to the point where I wanted to watch the Royal Ballet when it visited town, or go to the New York City Ballet, just to see people dancing the choreography flat out. Coming back to London I was interested to see how many of the new dancers here are concerned with dance and dance expression as such. In New York there are so many different kinds of work going on that it's almost impossible to make value judgements. (One of Britain's leading young choreographers talking to the author, on his return from two years of study with Merce Cunningham and others.)

Work is not divorceable from its social context or the predominant ideologies ... Dance needs to be seen in a wider context ... [it] is an energy booster which then needs focusing. A specialized language cuts you off from the people. (From a member of the X6 radical collective, trained at the Royal Ballet School and The Place.)

People have talked about making movement simpler, going back to natural forms, etc., but I would love to find a way of making it richer, more complicated, not necessarily going back to the beginning, but working with what has already formed my experience.' (An associate choreographer of the London Contemporary Dance Theatre.)

Similar observations are being made in every western centre that has nurtured a professional dance tradition – or, if this is not yet so, it soon will be. Because the new choreographers avoid obvious themes and narrative, they feel the need to communicate their aims verbally. In practice this may mean witty or peculiar titles for works, cerebral programme notes that contrast oddly with the simplicity of what the spectators actually watch. But there is no coercion involved in seeking out and holding an

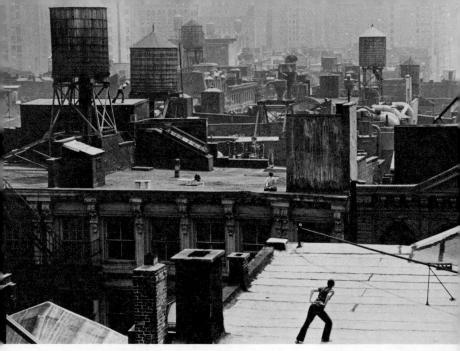

Trisha Brown's notorious roof-top dance, in Manhattan

audience. An open-air performance in a square would be designed to capture the passing attention of office workers in their lunch hour or, in an art gallery, the dances would be choreographed to complement the paintings on display. American experimentalists have set dancers in action along a line of roof tops and moved the audience from one location to another during the course of a single event. No one is astonished or upset if members of the public drop out or lose interest. Such a laissez-faire attitude makes an abrupt departure from the accepted rules of show business that have for so long dominated the performing arts.

There exists a middle range of contemporary groups which, although they do not choose to ignore the traditional rules, yet present more advanced works than are found within the mainstream. The majority of such companies are American, and led

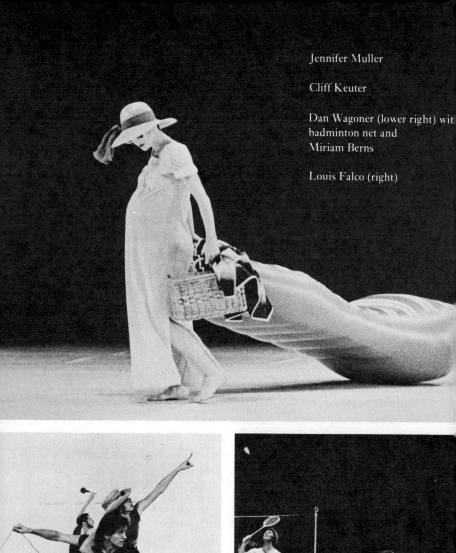

Jennifer Muller

Cliff Keuter

Dan Wagoner (lower right) wit
badminton net and
Miriam Berns

Louis Falco (right)

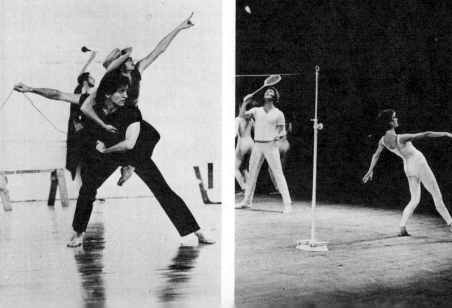

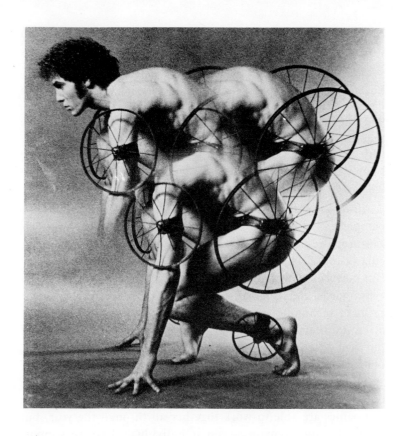

by a director-choreographer who dominates the repertory. They
have acquired the trappings of a full-time operation and
accepted the hardships of regular touring as well as the restric-
tion of performing the same works over and over again. They are
the most visible of all modern dance units, appearing in a variety
of theatres in many different countries. The spectrum ranges
from the established greats, like Graham Cunningham, Nikolais
and Taylor, through the zany, surprising, entertaining ensembles
of Louis Falco, Murray Louis, Pilobolus and Jennifer Muller to
the more challenging ones led by Trisha Brown, Douglas Dunn,
Cliff Keuter, Twyla Tharp and Dan Wagoner.

A Canadian mover, Margaret Dragu, wrote a wry prescription for such an undertaking:

Get a dance company kit – a business manager, a logo, an artistic director, a choreographer, a school, a performance season and some dancers – three females and two males. You can find dancers easily. They are in the audience. And they pretty much all look alike and think the same. They tend to be skinny, whiteanglosaxonprotestants, pretty, with skin as smooth and pale as the yoghurt that they always seem to be eating. They are conservative souls who enjoy repetition and domination.

Although nothing could be further from the truth with the companies led by the choreographers named above, Dragu has captured the essence of the many floating pick-up groups, particularly those which emerge from a dance academy or college. But performers with a Falco or a Tharp are separated from the avant-garde and the half-baked student companies by their brilliant technique and professional flexibility. The line-up is often multiracial and the choreographer will take advantage of physical differences among members. Group discipline is strict, but because the dancers often contribute to the choreography, and numbers are small, the atmosphere tends to be much more easy-going than in larger, establishment ensembles. Few of these companies are able to work together all through the year, but their allegiance remains, even if individuals have to support themselves by dancing with others or teaching for periods.

Twyla Tharp can be seen as the most potent symbol of this particular approach to modern dance. She has gone from being the darling of the avant-garde, so far-out that she fascinated and alienated critics and fans, to becoming something of a cult figure. Her distinctive, geometric hair bob, a long fringe obscuring her eyebrows, even became known as the 'Tharp cut' – a rare instance of experimental choreographer as a household name. In part, her immense popularity stems from creations for two major

Twyla Tharp with Ken Rinker in her televised work *Sue's Leg*

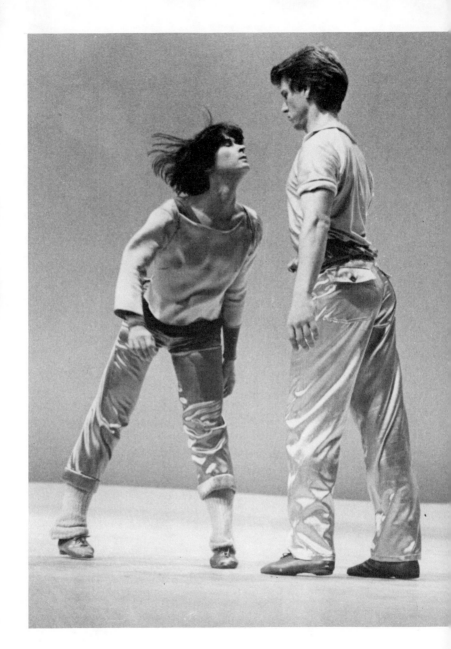

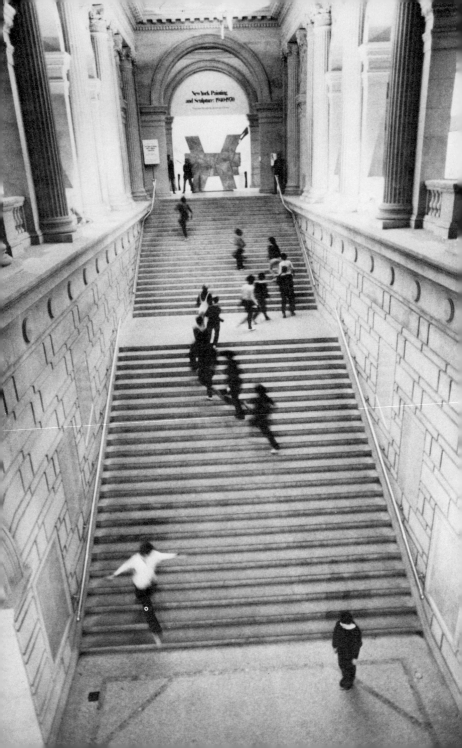

classical companies, the Joffrey and American Ballet Theatre, and her performances on television in works specially designed for the medium. Before 1971 she explored non-theatre spaces, mounting pieces in a gymnasium, libraries, museums and parks, and at one point suggested to New York authorities that she choreograph a number for police cadets to show 'the nature of control and its implementation' and help them 'ritualize certain hostilities, i.e. the wielding of a stick into the twirling of a baton'. (The proposal was rejected.) When her then all-woman company performed in a theatre, she might shift the audience on stage with the dancers, leaving the auditorium seats empty, or place a large box in the performing area so spectators could see only a segment of the action at any given moment.

During this period of exploration Tharp was evolving a unique style which combined fast, slick pop movements with the virtuosity of modern and ballet techniques. Russian star Mikhail Baryshnikov describes her approach in a book about his varied roles:

> As I began to work with her I found things very difficult technically. The body movement is often slightly off-balance – on purpose, of course – something completely foreign to my very straightforward classical way of moving ... In Twyla's work the body can switch direction in the middle of the beat for any given movement. She not only has these changes in the arc of each movement, as well as complicated variations, but the choreographic structure is very broad, all over the stage, and performed at top speed. As you are dancing you feel like a fish in the sand.

Intensely musical, Tharp has used jazz, blue grass, ragtime, rock, Haydn and Mozart, sometimes combining a modern composition with a baroque; and in her unaccompanied dance *The Fugue* the percussive boot stamps of the dancers weave intricate rhythms. (One British reviewer was convinced that he had heard an actual music score.) Her works have a driving

Tharp dancers on the stairs of the Metropolitan Museum of Art in New York

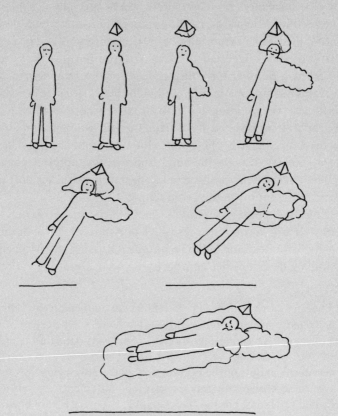

A PYRAMID OVER MY HEAD
A GOLDEN VEIL COMES TO COVER MY BODY AS
MY LEFT HAND BECOMES A BLUE CLOUD
I RISE AND FLOAT
MY HEAD RESTING ON MY CLOUD.

Remy Charlip

flow spiked with throwaway, deadpan humour that can look almost improvised, yet is tightly controlled and structured. Although she has achieved wide acceptance and acclaim, in her prickly independence and dictatorial attitude towards her creations she is something of a throwback to the tough-minded founders of modern dance. Yet in her willingness to try anything, even an ice number for skater John Curry, she most successfully represents the open-minded approach of some of the finest dancemakers of the day.

A French wit declared that there is no such thing as an avant-garde, only people lagging behind. With more than two thousand diverse dance performances reported in 1977 in Manhattan alone, and the erosion of demarcation lines between different techniques and styles, pigeon-holing is difficult; nothing in the arts is new, except technology, and everything has been tried before. But when you hear electronic music hum through the hallowed orchestra pit of the Royal Opera House, or note that the arch-rebel Merce Cunningham has been commissioned to mount a piece for the venerable Paris Opéra Ballet, you realize that the forces of creative experimentation are beginning to be accepted. The dancers operating on a shoe-string in lofts and church halls have made their mark, and the art form has been significantly enlivened by their contributions.

A unique way to create choreography: Remy Charlip's instructions for an 'airmail dance'. Anything goes? This illustration copyright © Remy Charlip.

Magazines, Books and Directories

Technical manuals and specialized academic publications are not included. Prices are generally in British sterling or American dollars, and paperback editions, where available, are mentioned.

These specialist book shops stock all or the majority of the titles listed below and provide a mailing service unless noted:

The Ballet Shop, a Dance Book Shop and Gallery, 1887 Broadway, New York, NY 10023, USA. No postal service.

Bookshop of Margareta Webber, 343 Little Collins Street, Melbourne 3000, Australia.

Dance Books, 9 Cecil Court, London WC2N 4EZ, UK. Publishes books and sends out lists of new books and additions to stock.

Drama Bookshop, 150 West 52nd Street, New York, NY 10019, USA.

La Danse, 14 Rue de Beaune, 75007 Paris, France.

Dance Mart, Box 48, Homecrest Station, Brooklyn, New York, NY 11229, USA. Postal service only. Catalogue available.

Library and Museum of the Performing Arts Sales Shop, 111 Amsterdam Avenue, New York, NY 10023.

GENERAL REFERENCE

The Concise Oxford Dictionary of Ballet, Horst Koegler, Oxford University Press, 1977.
This German critic's brief includes key figures in ethnic and modern dance, as well as classical ballet, sometimes with short bibliographies. Accurate and thorough.

The Encyclopedia of Dance and Ballet, edited by Mary Clarke and David Vaughan, Pitman Publishing, 1977.
Expensive but invaluable, with lavish illustrations (some in colour) and

contributions by a host of distinguished experts in different fields of dance. Includes long articles on subjects like design, the avant-garde and dance in film, which are particularly informative.

The Dance Horizon's Travel Guide to Six of the World's Dance Capitals, Sally and Eric Jacobson, Dance Horizons, New York, 1978 (paperback).
Useful directory of the main companies, theatres, schools, research centres, etc., of New York, Washington, London, Paris, Leningrad and Moscow.

MAGAZINES

Ballet Review, edited by Robert Cornfield and Nancy Reynolds. Quarterly. Subscription $30 per year plus $5 per volume postage outside the United States.
Wide-ranging, lengthy articles by working artists as well as by scholars and critics.
Address for subscriptions: Marcel Dekker Inc., PO Box 11305, Church Street Station, New York, NY 10249, USA.

Dance and Dancers, edited by Peter Williams. Monthly. 50p per issue; annual subscription £7.80 (US $15.60).
Long established, well-illustrated magazine with an international coverage that emphasizes dance in Britain and Europe. Stylishly written.
Address for subscriptions: Hansom Books, PO Box 294, 2 & 4 Old Pye Street, off Strutton Ground, Victoria Street, London SW1P 2LR, UK.

Dance Magazine, edited by William Como. Monthly. $2 per issue; annual subscription $18. (Add $3 per annum outside the USA.)
Encyclopedic coverage with American and international news reports plus long and short reviews, interviews and articles on all aspects of dance, and an educational directory. Level of writing is variable but an essential source of information.
Address for subscriptions: PO Box 960, Farmingdale, NY 11735, USA.

Dance in Canada, edited by Michael Crabb. Quarterly. $2 per issue; annual subscription $7.50 Canadian.

Lively journal with a range of contributors. The emphasis is on the Canadian scene. Bilingual (French and English).
Address for subscriptions: Dance in Canada Association, 100 Richmond East, Suite 325, Toronto, Ontario, Canada.

Dance Chronicle: studies in dance and related arts, edited by George Dorris and Jack Anderson. New publication; there will probably be four volumes per year. Subscription $16.25 per volume. Add $2.70 per volume for postage outside USA.
Address for subscription as for *Ballet Review*.

Dance Life, edited by David Lindner. Published quarterly. Single copy $2; subscription for three issues $5.50.
Well-illustrated journal with articles by well-known writers on most aspects of dance.
Address for subscriptions: Dance Life, Apt BA–1, 158 East 7th Street, New York, NY 10009, USA.

Dance Scope: a magazine of American dance, edited by Richard Lorber. Published semi-annually by the American Dance Guild. Single copy $2.50; annual subscription $8.50. Add $2.50 per year for postage outside USA.
Wide-ranging journal with good coverage of new and/or experimental dance.
Address for subscriptions: Dance Scope, 152 W 42nd St, Room 829, New York, NY 10036, USA.

Dans, published by The Dance Museum of Stockholm. Quarterly. Annual subscription: Europe outside Scandinavia and Finland 27 Swedish kr.; USA and Canada 36 Swedish kr.
Focus on Northern European dance but also covers major festivals and premières elsewhere. Bilingual in a Scandinavian language and English.
Address for subscriptions: Dans, PO Box 27 109, 102 52 Stockholm, Sweden.

Les Saisons de la Danse, edited by André-Phillipe Hérsin. Monthly. Single copy 7 francs.
French glossy which concentrates on the Paris scene.
Address for subscriptions: 3 rue des Petits-Carreaux, 75002 Paris, France.

Pour la Danse. Bi-monthly. Single copy 9 francs.
Well-illustrated and with a wider coverage than *Les Saisons de la Danse*.
Address for subscriptions: 36 rue Sainte, 13001 Marseille, France.

Chapter 1 : Mass Movements

Abe Peck, ed., *Dancing Madness*, Anchor Books, New York, 1976 (paperback).
A guide to current disco trends with illustrated expositions of some popular styles like the L A Hustle, Reggae and Salsa, plus a survey of seven decades of social dance.

Peter Buckingham, *Let's Dance*, Paddington Press, London, 1978.
Illustrated history of social, ballroom and folk dance.

Marshall and Jean Stearns, *Jazz Dance : the story of American vernacular dance*, Macmillan Company, New York; Collier-Macmillan Ltd, London, 1968.
Superb history, entertaining and well documented, with a selected list of films featuring jazz, tap and social dance plus a notation section of Afro-American dance styles. Now out of print but worth ordering from the library.

Arlene Croce, *The Fred Astaire and Ginger Rogers Book*, Vintage Books, 1977 (paperback).
Well-illustrated study in popular culture as exemplified by the careers of two famous American film-star dancers.

Belinda Quirey, with Steve Bradshaw and Ronald Smedley, *May I Have the Pleasure? the story of popular dancing*, British Broadcasting Corporation, 1976 (paperback).
Published to accompany a BBC television series of the same title, excellent illustrations, good section on rock dance.

Nik Cohn, *Awopbopaloobop Alopbamboom*, Paladin, 1970 (paperback).
Fast, funny, highly subjective survey of pop, including passing references to the dance crazes of different periods.

Curt Sachs, *World History of the Dance*, Norton, New York, 1963 (paperback).
Published in Germany under the title *Eine Weltgeschichte des Tanzes*.

Scholarly book by a distinguished ethnomusicologist, which discusses the evolution of dance and various social forms. Interesting but heavy.

Chapter 2: Training and Participation

Dance Magazine Annual and *Dance Magazine's Directory of Dance in Colleges and Universities*, both from Dance Magazine, 10 Columbus Circle, New York, NY 10019.

The annual is an exhaustive guide to artists and services, including professional associations of administrators, dance therapists, sources of reference materials, educational organizations, etc. Basically American focus but international information included. Essential.

The directory is a guide to dance in higher education, primarily in the USA. The Dance Magazine postal service for books and historic portfolios operates from the same address.

Dancing Times, edited by Mary Clarke. Monthly. 40p per issue; £5.50 annual subscription (US $12.75).

Some review coverage and general articles on dance with a regular educational section. Good for addresses of examining boards, schools, etc., mainly in Britain but with some international data. Runs a book service which includes suggested titles for GCE exams and an information service on teaching.

Address for subscriptions and book service: 18 Hand Court, High Holborn, London WC1 1V6JF, UK. Subscription agent in North America: Sportshelf, PO Box 634, New Rochelle, New York, USA.

Dance collection, New York Public Library, Performing Arts Research Center, Lincoln Center, 111 Amsterdam Avenue, New York, NY 10023, USA (Curator: Genevieve Oswald).

Dansmuseum, PO Box 27 109, 102 52 Stockholm, Sweden (Director: Bengt Hager).

Growth of Dance in America (*Arts in Society*, vol. 13, no. 2, Summer-Fall 1976, paperback). Can be ordered from Arts in Society, University of Wisconsin, Room 728, Lowell Hall, 610 Langdon Street, Madison, Wisconsin 53706, USA.

Interesting collection of essays on topics like dance literacy and dance in academe, and a symposium: 'Training the dancer'.

Richard Cornell and Mary Lewis Hansen, *Exploring Dance Careers: A Student Guidebook*, US Government Printing Office, Washington, 1976 (paperback).

Hilary Cartwright, *Dancing for a Living: a career in the world of dance*, Educational Explorers Ltd, Reading, UK, 1974.
Primarily a guide to professional ballet careers, although modern dance is mentioned in passing.

Walter Terry, *Career for the '70s; Dance*, Crowell-Collier Press, New York; Collier-Macmillan Ltd, London, 1971.

Chapter 3: Modern Dance – Pioneers and Popularizers

Isadora Duncan, *My Life*, Gollancz, London, 1966.
Autobiography ending with the dancer's departure for Russia in 1921.

Ilya Ilyitch Schneider, *Isadora Duncan: the Russian years*, MacDonald, London, 1968.
An account of Duncan's adventures in Russia, 1921–6.

Don McDonagh, *Martha Graham: a biography*, David & Charles, London, 1974; Popular Library, New York, 1975 (paperback). Illustrated.

Walter Terry, *Frontiers of Dance: the life of Martha Graham*, Thomas Y. Crowell, New York, 1975.
A young person's version, part of the 'Women of America' series. Illustrated.

Doris Humphrey, *The Art of Making Dances*, Holt, Rinehart & Winston, New York, 1959; Grove Press, New York, 1962 (paperback). Illustrated. A great artist's credo, written simply and with intelligence and charm.

Selma Jeanne Cohen, *Doris Humphrey: an artist first*, Wesleyan University Press, Connecticut, 1972. Illustrated.

Olga Maynard, *American Modern Dancers: the pioneers*, Little, Brown & Co., Boston, Toronto, 1965.
Short biographical chapters on Duncan, Wigman, St Denis, Shawn, Humphrey, etc.

Joseph H. Mazo, *Prime Movers: the makers of modern dance in America*, William Morrow & Co., New York, 1977.
Biographical sketches and critical analysis of the contributions of Fuller, Duncan, St Denis, Shawn, Humphrey, Graham, Cunningham, Nikolais, Ailey, Taylor and Tharp. Includes discussion of the avant-garde. Illustrated.

James Klosty, ed., *Merce Cunningham*, E. P. Dutton & Co., New York, 1975 (paperback).
Beautiful photographs by the editor, who has collected essays on Cunningham from some of his most important collaborators. Essential.

Richard Kostelanetz, ed., *John Cage*, Allen Lane, 1971 (paperback, 1974).

Selma Jeanne Cohen, ed., *The Modern Dance: seven statements of belief*, Wesleyan University Press, Connecticut, 1966 (paperback, 1969).
Articles by choreographers Limon, Nikolais, Taylor, etc.

Don McDonagh, *The Complete Guide to Modern Dance*, Doubleday, New York, 1976; Popular Library, New York, 1977 (paperback).
The work of more than 100 American modernists is examined. Invaluable for reference, albeit incomplete.

Don McDonagh, *The Rise and Fall and Rise of Modern Dance*, Dutton, New York, 1970; Mentor, New American Library, New York, 1971 (paperback).
A chattier, less exhaustive early model of the title above, including a brief history and analysing the contributions of key choreographers.

Walter Terry, *The Dance in America*, Harper & Row, revised edition, 1971.
American ballet is covered but the emphasis is firmly, and informatively, on contemporary and ethnic dance, with some discussion of dance education, notation, dance in musicals and film etc. Illustrated.

Merce Cunningham, edited by Frances Starr, *Changes: notes on choreography*, Something Else Press, New York, 1968.
A confusing, exhilarating look into Cunningham's working notebooks. Illustrated.

Moira Hodgson, *Quintet: Five American Dance Companies*, Gage, New York, 1976.
An account of the ensembles directed by Alvin Ailey, Merce Cunningham, Elliot Feld (modern ballet), Paul Taylor and the Dance Theater of Harlem.

Chapter 4: Classical Ballet: The Mainstream

BIOGRAPHIES AND AUTOBIOGRAPHIES
Ninette de Valois, *Come Dance with Me*, Dance Books Ltd, London, 1978.
Memoirs by the founder of Britain's Royal Ballet.

Romola Nijinsky, *Nijinsky*, Sphere Books, London, 1970 (paperback).
Emotional biography by the late dancer's wife.

Richard Buckle, *Nijinsky*, Simon & Schuster, New York, 1971.
Illustrated.
Definitive biography by the British critic.

Keith Money, *John Curry*, Michael Joseph, London, 1978.
Money provides some stunning photographs and an introduction; Curry writes honestly of his skating experiences and love of dance. Expensive.

V. Svetloff, *Anna Pavlova*, Dover Publications, New York, 1974 (large paperback).

Margot Fonteyn: Autobiography, W. H. Allen, London, 1975; A. Knopf, New York, 1976; Warner Books, New York, 1977 (paperback).

Bernard Taper, *Balanchine*, Collier-Macmillan, New York, revised edition 1975 (paperback).

Agnes de Mille, *Speak to Me, Dance with Me*, Popular Library, New York, 1973 (paperback).
Entertaining and well written reminiscences of this American choreographer's period with the Ballet Rambert in England.

Marie Rambert, *Quicksilver, an Autobiography*, Macmillan, London, 1972.
Delightful book by the founder of the Ballet Rambert.

Baryshnikov at Work: Mikhail Baryshnikov discusses his roles, text edited and introduced by Charles Engell France, photographs by Martha Swope, Adam & Charles Black, London, 1977; A. Knopf, New York, 1977.
Large, beautiful, expensive volume with the Russian dancer providing perceptive commentary on the wide range of roles he has interpreted during his meteoric career.

John Percival, *Nureyev: aspects of the dancer*, Faber & Faber, London, 1975.
Illustrated, well-documented, but rather uncritical study of the super-star.

GENERAL HISTORY

Peter Brinson and Clement Crisp, *Ballet for All*, David & Charles, revised ed., 1971; Pan Books, London, 1970 (paperback).
Detailed analysis of more than one hundred important ballets, with a linking historical narrative.

Mary Clarke and Clement Crisp, *Making a Ballet*, Studio Vista, London, 1974.
A survey of the processes by which choreographers create a ballet. Illustrated.

Nancy Reynolds, *Repertory in Review: Forty Years of the New York City Ballet*, Dial Press, New York, 1977.
Comprehensive history of a major company with detailed descriptions of more than 200 ballets created by Balanchine and others. Illustrated.

Ian Woodward, *Ballet*, Hodder and Stoughton (Teach Yourself Books), 1977 (paperback). General introduction plus an appendix containing who's who, ballet definitions, the basic repertory, etc.

Joan Lawson, *The Story of Ballet*, Ward Lock, London, 1976.
A young person's history encompassing some discussion of technique and training. Profusely illustrated.

Joan Lawson, *Dance Data 1*, Two Charts: 'The Development of Classical Ballet' and 'A Chart for the History of Dance in Society and in the Theatre as Ballet', Dance Horizons, New York, 1978.
Clear, graphic booklet compiled for students at Britain's Royal Ballet School. Inexpensive.

Natalia Roslavleva, *Era of the Russian Ballet*, Gollancz, London, 1966.
Illustrated history from 1770 to 1965.

Rudi Van Danzig and others, *Ballet and Modern Dance*, Octopus Books, London, 1974.
Short, lavishly illustrated chapters on major dance companies and choreographers. Popular introduction.

Selma Jeanne Cohen, ed., *Dance as a Theatre Art: source readings in dance history from 1581 to the present*, Dodd, Mead & Co., New York, 1974 (paperback).
Absorbing anthology with original writings by major modern choreographers as well as by ballet figures.

Jack Anderson, *Dance*, Newsweek Books, New York, 1974.
Stylishly written, informative history with good illustrations. Includes contemporary dance.

Alexander Bland, *A History of Ballet and Dance*, Barrie & Jenkins, London, 1976.
Off-putting cover photo of Fonteyn and Nureyev but beautifully illustrated inside, with lots of colour plates. Brisk, chatty prose with a particularly interesting chapter on design and scenic effects. Basically a summary of western theatre dance, the emphasis being placed on classical ballet.

Richard Philp and Mary Whitney, *Danseur: the Male in Ballet*, McGraw-Hill, New York, 1977.
Expensive, lavishly illustrated history of the male classical dancer.

John Percival, *The World of Diaghilev*, Studio Vista, London, 1971 (hardback and paperback).
Picture survey of the famous director and his colleagues. Very basic.

Lincoln Kirstein, *Movement and Metaphor*, Pitman Publishing, London; Praeger Publishers, New York, 1970.
Subtitled 'Four Centuries of Ballet'; the author, co-founder of the New York City Ballet, surveys five basic elements of theatrical dance and analyses fifty seminal works.

David Vaughan, *Sir Frederick Ashton and His Ballets*, Adam & Charles Black, London, 1977.
Definitive survey of the great British choreographer's creations.

W. G. Raffe, comp., *Dictionary of the Dance*, A. S. Barnes & Co., New York; Thomas Yoseloff Ltd, London, 1964.
Definitions and explanations of traditional dance forms from more than one hundred different countries. Rather expensive.

Geoffrey Gorer, *Africa Dances*, Faber & Faber, London, 1935.
Now out of print and out of date but a marvellously vivid description of the role of dance in the life of West Africans. Worth searching for in libraries.

Lynne Fauley Emery, *Black Dance in the United States from 1619 to 1970*, Mayfield Publishing, Palo Alto, California, 1972.
Disgracefully, this is already out of print but it is such an invaluable historical record of the evolution of western, black dance that it should be obtainable from any serious library.

Joseph Mazo, *The Alvin Ailey American Dance Theater*, William Morrow & Co., New York, 1978 (paperback).
Photographs by Susan Cook and a short, interesting introduction to the work of this attractive company.

D. E. Pohren, *The Art of Flamenco*, The Society of Spanish Studies, Sevilla, 1962.

Anna Ivanova, *The Dancing Spaniards*, John Baker, London, 1970.
Comprehensive account of the development and current difficulties of Spanish dance.

Clifford Jones and Betty True Jones, *Kathakali : an introduction to the dance-drama of Kerala*, Theatre Arts Books, New York, 1970 (paperback).
Popular introduction to this complex, ancient art-form with helpful illustrations.

Kapila Vatsyayan, *Indian Classical Dance*, Ministry of Information and Broadcasting, New Delhi, 1974.
Interesting, technical analysis of the different styles. Particularly strong on comparisons among the various traditions of dance.

Rina Singha and Reginald Massey, *Indian Dances : their history and growth*, Faber & Faber, London, 1967.

Now slightly out of date concerning the revival of certain styles, but a good general introduction. Illustrated.

Ira Friedlander, *The Whirling Dervishes*, Wildwood House Ltd, London, 1975 (hardback and paperback).
Fascinating photo study with informative text about the Sufi order.

Ted Petrides, *Greek Dances*, Lycabettus Press, Athens, 1975 (paperback).
A popular guide, with technical drawings, to the main folk dances of Greece.

Chapter 6: Alternative Dance

MAGAZINES

As well as those mentioned in the General Reference section, of which the American publications *Dance Magazine* and *Dance Scope* and the British *Dance and Dancers* give the most space to experimental work, there is a new journal which concentrates entirely on this area:
New Dance. Quarterly. 50p per issue, £2.50 annual subscription, £4.00 airmail subscription to USA and Canada.
Very basically (i.e. cheaply) produced magazine, edited by a dance collective. Contains articles and reviews about alternative movers in Britain, with occasional pieces about similar activities elsewhere.
Address for subscriptions: X6 Dance Space, Butler's Wharf, Lafone St, London SE1, UK.

Soho Weekly News and *Village Voice*, newspapers published every week in New York; both contain extensive coverage (reviews, interviews and listings) of alternative dance. *Time Out* magazine provides a similar service in London.

COLLECTIONS

The two surveys by Don McDonagh mentioned in the reading list for Chapter Three both contain valuable material on experimental dance. Otherwise, the best general guides are collected reviews by American dance critics Arlene Croce, Jill Johnston, Deborah Jowitt and Marcia B. Siegel, which cover aspects of the New York avant-garde in considerable detail:

Jill Johnston, *Marmalade Me*, Dutton, New York, 1971 (paperback). Most of these essays appeared in *Village Voice* between 1960 and 1970, and provide a fascinating historical survey of the early days of the Judson Dance Theatre by a writer who was herself closely involved in the movement.

Deborah Jowitt, *Dance Beat: Selected Views and Reviews, 1967–1976*, Marcel Dekker, New York, 1977 (paperback).
Perceptive essays by Johnston's successor on *Village Voice*.

Marcia B. Siegel, *At the Vanishing Point: a critic looks at dance*, Dutton, New York, 1972; Saturday Review Press, New York, 1973 (paperback).

Marcia B. Siegel, *Watching the Dance Go By*, Houghton Mifflin Co., Boston, 1977 (paperback).
Excellent summary of the avant-garde.

John Cage, *M: Writings, 1967–72*, Calder, 1973; Calder & Boyars, 1976 (paperback); *Silence*, Calder, 1968; Calder, 1973 (paperback); *A Year from Monday*, Calder, 1968; Calder, 1972 (paperback).
Collected writings and lectures by the iconoclastic composer, long-time collaborator with Merce Cunningham.

Simone Forti, *Handbook in Motion*, Nova Scotia College of Art and Design, Halifax, 1974. Illustrated.
Subjective theories by a leading exponent of performance art.

Yvonne Rainer, *Work 1961–73*, Nova Scotia College of Art and Design, Halifax, 1974.
A founder of the Judson Dance Theatre discusses her approach.

Arlene Croce, *Afterimages*, Afred A. Knopf, New York, 1978.
The founder and editor of *Ballet Review*, currently dance critic for the *New Yorker*, has assembled a pungent selection of articles covering the last decade of American dance.

Useful Addresses

FOR TRAINING INFORMATION

The *Dance Magazine Annual* and the *Dance Horizons Travel Guide to Six of the World's Dance Capitals* both contains addresses of organizations which will supply information about teachers and schools. As the majority of the *Annual*'s addresses are in the United States of America, some contacts in other English-speaking countries are given below.

It must be stressed that many of the best teachers are private, and that it is impossible to list particular schools, however well-established. The majority of the associations below are concerned with classical ballet, because individualistic modern dance teachers generally avoid representative associations. Specialist magazines remain the best guide to details of training opportunities.

British Ballet Organization, Woolborough House, 39 Londsdale Rd, London SW1 3 9JP.
Imperial Society of Teachers of Dancing, 70 Gloucester Place, London W1H 4J.
International Dance Teachers Association, 76 Bennett Road, Brighton, BN2 5JL, England.
Royal Academy of Dancing, 48 Vicarage Crescent, London SW11 3LT.
   RAD Branches in
   Australia: 254 George St, Sydney 2000.
   Canada: 209/3050 Yonge St, Toronto, Ontario M4N 2K4.
   New Zealand: CPO Box 857, Wellington.
   USA: 8 College Avenue, Upper Montclair, New Jersey 07043.
Society of Russian Style Ballet, Mrs Burns, 65 Tiverton Rd, Potters Bar, Herts., England.
   Branch in Canada: Marijan Bayer, 1875 Leslie St, Unit 24, Don Mills, Ontario.
Dance in Canada Association, 100 Richmond East, Suite 325, Toronto, Ontario.

Acknowledgements

Special thanks to Cornelia Bach, the picture researcher for *Time Out* magazine who made available the magazine's extensive photo archives and loaned several illustrations for this book. Also, warmest thanks to David Leonard of Dance Books in London, who gave invaluable advice on which titles should be included in the reference section. Press officers of several British dance companies, notably Tony Barlow of London Festival Ballet, Janet Judd of the Royal Ballet, Olivia Maxwell of the London Contemporary Dance Theatre and Seona Reid of Ballet Rambert, were particularly helpful in supplying me with photographic and research material, as was David Palmer, the press representative for several major ballet companies. Sarah Woodcock of the Theatre Museum in the Victoria and Albert Museum kindly found the early photo of Martha Graham, and Ton Leenhouts of the Nederlands Dans Theatre provided an extensive collection of photos of his own company. Another cooperative Dutch publicist is Dick Hendricks of the National Ballet. And in New York, the staff of the Performing Arts Services, the Merce Cunningham Foundation, the press office of the Public Broadcasting Station, and Norma McLain Stoop and Tobi Tobias of *Dance Magazine* all provided assistance. My friend Ellis Rothenberg helped me sort out the mass of photographic material, some of which had been stored under beds but survived intact.

The author and publishers would also like to thank the following for permission to reproduce illustrative material. COMPANIES AND THEATRES: Alvin Ailey American Dance Theatre for page 67 *below* (photo: Ken Duncan) and page 126; The Australian Ballet for page 123 *below left* (photo: David Parker); Béjart's Ballet for page 120 (photo: Kayaert); Bolshoi Ballet for page 41 *above*; Trisha Brown's Company for page 47 *below* (photo: Jack Mitchell) and 149 *middle*; National Ballet of Canada for page 106 *below*; Ballet Internacional de Caracas for page 123 *above left* (photo: Ricardo Armas); The Cullberg Ballet for page 83 *above*; Merce Cunningham and Dance Company for page 79 *above* (photo: Penny Brogden), and 79 *below* (photo: Herb Migdoll); Royal Danish Ballet (photo: John R. Johnson) for page 111 *left*; Dutch National Ballet for page 103 *above* (photo: Jorge Fatauros) and 122 *above right*;

Louis Falco Dance Company for page 161; Martha Graham Center for Contemporary Dance for page 73; Dance Theatre of Harlem for page 129 (photo: Marbeth); The Joffrey Ballet for page 123 *above right*; Korean National Dance Company for page 140 *below*; MAAS for page 134; Nederlands Dans Theater for page 80 *above* (photo: Tony Van Muden) and 80 *below* (photo: Sven Ulsa); New York City Ballet for pages 2–3 and 41 *above*; Nikolais Dance Theatre for page 79 *below* (photo: P. Bertheldt); Roland Petit's Ballets de Marseille for page 123 *below right*; Pilobolus Dance Theatre for page 153 *below left* and *right*; Ballet Rambert for pages 45 *above* and *below* and 81 *above* (photo: Charles Milligan); Royal Ballet for pages 107 *above* (photo: Reg Wilson) and 119; Sadler's Wells Theatre for pages 122 *below right*, 141 *below*, 145 *below* and 153 *above*; Janet Smith for page 157 *above left*; National Dance Company of Spain for page 144 *left* (photo: Magi); The Paul Taylor Dance Foundation for page 77; Twyla Tharp Dance Foundation for page 164 (photo: James Klotsty); Anne Wyman Dance Theatre for page 88.

PHOTOGRAPHERS: S. A. Ashaye and Abey Photoservice for page 133; Nobby Clark for page 144 *right*; Anthony Crickmay for page 46 *above* and *below*, 47 *above*, 82 *below*, 84, 107 *above*, 108 *below*, 113 *above left* and 122 *above left* and *below left*; Alan Cunliffe for page 130; Pierre Farge for page 131 *left*; Mark Gamon for page 151; Gilda Grillo for page 131 *right*; Robert Hartman for page 87; Shuhei Iwamoto for page 132; Camilla Jessel for page 39; Helen Leoussi for pages 156 *above left* and 156 *below*; Babette Mangolte for page 159; Robert Morgan for page 37; Mula and Haramaty for page 83 *below*; Christopher Schwarz for page 146; Leslie E. Spatt for page 117; Martha Swope for pages 73 *middle*, 103 *below*, 111 *below right*, 114, and 128; Pat Ward for page 55, 56 and 147 *above*; Mike Wells for page 108 *above*; Geoff White for pages 156 *above right* and 157 *below*; OTHERS: BBC for page 36, 79 *above* and 113 *above right*; Camera Press for pages 12, 18 and 23 *below*; page 166 © Remy Charlip; International Freelance Library for page 141 *above* (photo: Mark Rusher); Keystone Press Agency for page 16 *left* and *right*, 23 *above* and 32; Kobal Collection for page 21; London Features International for page 24 (photo: Michael Putland); London Weekend Television for pages 85 and 106 *above*; The Lost and Foundation for the Arts for page 160 *above* (photo: Jorge Fatauros); Raymond Mander and Jo Mitchison Theatre Collection for page 70 *above* and *below*, and 71 *above*; Radio Times Hulton Picture Library for page 14; *Time Out* for page 19, 25 *above* (photo: Sebastian Izzard), 25 *below* (photo: Alf Fox) 28, 29 (photo: Chris Horler), 31 and 34 *below* (photo: Aubrey Dewar); 34 *above* (photo: Walt Davidson) 102 *left* and *right* and 145 *above*; Theatre Museum, Victoria and Albert Museum for page 73 *above* (photo: Ira D. Schwarz); WNET/PBS for page 115 and 163.

Index

185